Investing in Children's Mental Health

Investing in Children's Mental Health

DANIEL EISENBERG AND
RAMESH RAGHAVAN

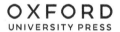
OXFORD
UNIVERSITY PRESS

OXFORD
UNIVERSITY PRESS

Oxford University Press is a department of the University of Oxford. It furthers
the University's objective of excellence in research, scholarship, and education
by publishing worldwide. Oxford is a registered trade mark of Oxford University
Press in the UK and certain other countries.

Published in the United States of America by Oxford University Press
198 Madison Avenue, New York, NY 10016, United States of America.

© Oxford University Press 2024

Library of Congress Cataloging-in-Publication Data
Names: Eisenberg, Daniel (Of Fielding School of Public Health), author. |
Raghavan, Ramesh, author.
Title: Investing in children's mental health / Daniel Eisenberg and
Ramesh Raghavan.
Description: New York, NY : Oxford University Press, [2024] |
Includes bibliographical references and index.
Identifiers: LCCN 2023032471 (print) | LCCN 2023032472 (ebook) |
ISBN 9780190942014 (paperback) | ISBN 9780190942038 (epub) |
ISBN 9780190942045 (online)
Subjects: MESH: Mental Health | Child | Adolescent | Mental Health Services |
Cost-Benefit Analysis
Classification: LCC RJ499.3 (print) | LCC RJ499.3 (ebook) |
NLM WS 105.5.M3 | DDC 618.9289–dc23/eng/20230908
LC record available at https://lccn.loc.gov/2023032471
LC ebook record available at https://lccn.loc.gov/2023032472

DOI: 10.1093/oso/9780190942014.001.0001

Printed by Marquis Book Printing, Canada

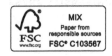

Contents

Introduction: Scope and Purpose of this Book   1

1. What Does It Mean to Invest in Children's Mental
   Health?   8

2. Overview of Current Evidence and Practice   18

3. Home Visiting Programs   37

4. Parent Training Programs   55

5. School-Based Social-Emotional Learning (SEL)
   Programs   70

6. Multisystemic Therapy: The Fluorescent Light Bulb
   Not Everyone Is Using   86

7. Communities That Care   102

8. Lessons Learned and Remaining Questions   114

9. A Path toward Better Investments   131

Index   151

Acknowledgments

This book would not have been possible without the many people who generously shared their experiences and wisdom in the conversations, interviews, and site visits we conducted. These individuals are practitioners, administrators, policymakers, and scholars, and all helped us to better understand the issues, deepen our thinking, and make our work more approachable and relevant. While they are too numerous to list here, many are mentioned in the chapters throughout the book. We continue to be inspired by their collective passion and commitment to support children and youth mental health. They make us optimistic that we can meet the challenges laid out in this book.

We thank the many mentors and colleagues who have encouraged and supported our work over the course of our careers to date. We also thank the acquisitions, editorial, and production teams at Oxford University Press for their hard work to produce this book; working with them has been a pleasure.

On a personal note, Daniel thanks his family for their unwavering support; they include his wife (Martha), their two children (Eve and Ella), his parents (Hélène and Robert), and his siblings (Nina, Sarah, and Louis). Ramesh thanks his wife (Sujatha) for her forbearance and support.

The two of us (Daniel and Ramesh) were professional friends who had read, and respected, each other's work for many years before we began writing this book. We are grateful for the opportunity to have worked on this project together, and we have learned a lot from each other. We believe that harmonious collaborations like this are needed on a much greater scale to address the complex challenge of improving children's mental health in the United States and beyond.

Introduction

Scope and Purpose of this Book

In the United States and many other countries, we are living in the midst of public health success stories, despite the recent COVID-19 pandemic. Over the past 50 years, mortality due to cardiovascular disease has decreased dramatically (Mensah et al., 2017), and cancer-related mortality has also fallen substantially (Siegel et al., 2018). Even with the well-known inefficiencies of the U.S. healthcare system, the general trend has been toward healthier and longer lives.

The successes of public health and medicine have not been universal, unfortunately, and this is particularly true for mental health conditions. Individuals with a mental disorder die on average 8.2 years younger than others (Druss et al., 2011). People who receive care for a mental disorder in the public health care system have higher death rates, and die at much younger ages, when compared with those without mental disorders (Colton & Manderscheid, 2006).

Children and adolescents who have a mental disorder are among the most vulnerable of all young people. Among families reporting a need, approximately half of children receive any mental health care, let alone high-quality and evidence-based care, and access to care is especially low for families of color and those living in poverty (Lu, 2017). The challenge is not just about access to treatment, however. There are also opportunities to prevent mental disorders before they emerge and progress to more severe levels, but such

Investing in Children's Mental Health. Daniel Eisenberg and Ramesh Raghavan, Oxford University Press.
© Oxford University Press 2024. DOI: 10.1093/oso/9780190942014.003.0001

prevention efforts are scattered and do not reach most children and families.

This book aims to help push forward our society's thinking and actions regarding children's mental health. In particular, we address three interrelated questions:

1. What are some of the best available investments to improve the mental health of children and adolescents in the United States?
2. To what extent are these investments being made?
3. What can practitioners, child-serving organizations, policy-makers, and other stakeholders do in order to promote such investments?

You might already be convinced of the importance of asking and answering these questions. But just to be sure, consider the following facts. Mental and behavioral health conditions inflict by far the most significant burden of disease, of any class of health conditions, among children and adolescents in the United States and other higher income countries (Erskine et al., 2015). Recent data indicate that we are going in the wrong direction, with rising depression, anxiety, and suicide risk among children and adolescents (Twenge et al., 2019). These challenges become even greater when we consider the rapidly evolving needs as children develop and mature, layered on top of the relentless societal changes driven by shifting culture and technology.

As important as they are, the questions posed in this book have not been adequately answered. One reason is that we are rarely even *asking* the questions, particularly in the United States. Our decentralized systems of healthcare, public health, and social services do not force our policymakers and other community leaders to address these questions in a unified, holistic manner. Even when we do ask the questions, it is easy to become discouraged or sidetracked by the complexity of arriving at answers. The evidence and data are enormously complicated and far from complete. In this book, we cannot claim to provide definitive answers ourselves; rather, our more modest objective is to bring these questions to the fore and offer initial observations that can set us on a clearer path toward productive solutions.

How We Approach Each Question

What are the best available investments? On a broad level, we provide a synthesis of currently available evidence and data, which are summarized in Chapter 2. This synthesis is facilitated by databases and meta-analyses that have already been carefully curated and conducted by other research groups, such as the Blueprints Program for Healthy Youth Development and the Washington State Institute for Public Policy. On a more in-depth level, we provide a series of case studies in Chapters 3–7 featuring a variety of mental health and behavioral programs that appear to be strong investments. We compiled these case studies through a synthesis of research and data from publicly available articles and reports, as well as our original interviews with program developers, practitioners who are implementing the programs in various communities across the United States, and other stakeholders and experts.

To what degree are these best available investments actually being made? In the broad overview of potential investments in Chapter 2, we stitch together data regarding the national penetration of programs with the strongest evidence of effectiveness and cost-effectiveness. These data illustrate that very few of the best investments have achieved widespread reach, whereas some questionable investments have. In other words, as a society we are failing systematically to make the best investments in children's mental health. The case studies in Chapters 3–7 provide a deeper look at the degree and nature of investments for specific types of programs.

What can we all do to promote best investments? In the final chapters of the book (Chapters 8–9), we distill themes and conclusions from these case studies, as well as the broader research and data. Our focus is on the primary factors that inhibit or facilitate making the best investments in children's mental health. We discuss implications and recommendations for a variety of audiences who could potentially promote, support, or implement such investments.

Perspectives of the Authors

This book was motivated by two recurrent observations in our research and discussions with policymakers and practitioners: First, there is a large and increasing number of excellent investments that can be made in children's mental health, and second, these investments are not generally being made adequately or successfully. If you work in an area related to children's mental health, you have probably made similar observations. We believe this gap points to one of the most important opportunities to improve the well-being of children and society more broadly. Thus, we feel compelled to examine and document the gap carefully and help make sense of how to address it most effectively as a society.

The two of us are coming at the topic from different and complementary paths. One of us, Daniel Eisenberg, started with the field of economics, drawn to its rigorous approach to grappling with social policy questions. Economics provides a unified, quantitative framework for identifying and evaluating opportunities for improving societal well-being. The framework has inevitable limitations, such as simplifying assumptions that are not realistic in every context, but it provides a transparent and cohesive way to evaluate social policy questions and consider the conclusions alongside the limitations of the analysis. Daniel has also been in the field of public health throughout his career as a professor; the public health perspective emphasizes factors beyond healthcare, such as social and economic stressors and preventive interventions, all of which are important for children's mental health. Although the mental health of young people has not traditionally been a core topic in economics or public health, the intersection of these subjects is natural and fruitful; they are all closely linked to the overall well-being and prosperity of societies.

Ramesh Raghavan, by contrast, started in the field of medicine and psychiatry, attracted by its direct and practical potential to improve human well-being. He then gained expertise in health services and policy research. His research has focused largely on understanding and improving factors that increase access to and improve quality of mental health services for vulnerable child populations. Such factors include financial mechanisms such as the Medicaid insurance program and organizational factors among providers and healthcare systems. He has been closely involved in the development and application of implementation science—which examines why and how programs and interventions can be successfully adopted, deployed, and sustained by organizations and communities. Ramesh has also developed a line of research on conceptualizing and measuring children's well-being. Thus, together we bring a multidisciplinary perspective rooted in economics, public health, medicine, and implementation science, among other fields.

What This Book Offers to Various Audiences

This book aims to be useful to several different audiences, including decision makers (policymakers, administrators, and other community and organizational leaders), practitioners (direct service professionals in mental health, education, and other fields), scholars (researchers and students), and concerned citizens (parents, other caregivers, and others interested in children's and societal well-being).

For decision makers, such as policymakers and administrators, the book provides a broad overview of investments to consider funding and implementing, as well as more detailed information about several specific investments with particularly strong evidence. These leaders might also find the book useful for informing their general thinking and processes by which they evaluate what makes a good investment and how to implement it successfully. Thus, our hope is that the book will help decision makers identify specific investment strategies and promote deliberate, well-informed decision and implementation processes more generally.

For practitioners such as mental health professionals and teachers, the book offers information about specific programs, as well as general types of programs, that they might want to consider promoting or providing in their local communities. This audience might also find ideas and strategies for *how* to advocate and implement such programs more effectively.

For scholars such as researchers and students, the book offers a general framework for addressing the questions posed by the book. This framework might be useful for these scholars in their own investigation of similar or related topics. The book also provides an overview of available data and research regarding the best investments in children's mental health. We hope that scholars will increase their appreciation of and attention to the large and important gaps that remain in our knowledge in this area. These questions require far more talent, time, and energy from the scholarly community.

Finally, for concerned citizens such as parents, other caregivers, and perhaps young people themselves, we hope to inspire a fuller appreciation for the opportunities we are missing—as a society and as communities, families, and individuals—to improve children's mental health and well-being. Although we describe many reasons to be concerned about the current situation, we hope that our readers will feel more motivated and optimistic about the possibilities for improvement. More practically, concerned citizens will find ideas for programs and investments to advocate for in our communities, and strategies for doing so effectively.

References

Colton, C. W., & Manderscheid, R. W. (2006). Congruencies in increased mortality rates, years of potential life lost, and causes of death among public mental health clients in eight states. *Preventing Chronic Disease, 3*(2), 1–14.

Druss, B. G., Zhao, L., Von Esenwein, S., Morrato, E. H., & Marcus, S. C. (2011). Understanding excess mortality in persons with mental illness: 17-year follow up of a nationally representative US survey. *Medical Care, 49*(6), 599–604.

Erskine, H., Moffitt, T. E., Copeland, W., Costello, E., Ferrari, A., Patton, G., Degenhardt, L., Vos, T., Whiteford, H., & Scott, J. (2015). A heavy burden on young minds: The global burden of mental and substance use disorders in children and youth. *Psychological Medicine, 45*(7), 1551–1563.

Lu, W. (2017). Child and adolescent mental disorders and health care disparities: Results from the National Survey of Children's Health, 2011–2012. *Journal of Health Care for the Poor and Underserved, 28*(3), 988–1011.

Mensah, G. A., Wei, G. S., Sorlie, P. D., Fine, L. J., Rosenberg, Y., Kaufmann, P. G., Mussolino, M. E., Hsu, L. L., Addou, E., & Engelgau, M. M. (2017). Decline in cardiovascular mortality: Possible causes and implications. *Circulation Research, 120*(2), 366–380.

Siegel, R. L., Jemal, A., Wender, R. C., Gansler, T., Ma, J., & Brawley, O. W. (2018). An assessment of progress in cancer control. *CA: A Cancer Journal for Clinicians, 68*(5), 329–339.

Twenge, J. M., Cooper, A. B., Joiner, T. E., Duffy, M. E., & Binau, S. G. (2019). Age, period, and cohort trends in mood disorder indicators and suicide-related outcomes in a nationally representative dataset, 2005–2017. *Journal of Abnormal Psychology, 128*(3), 185–199.

1

What Does It Mean to Invest in Children's Mental Health?

Imagine an elementary school where the principal and her team are considering how to support their children's social and mental health more effectively. They are wary of distracting from the core educational mission of the school, and they do not have a lot of extra resources and staff time. They recognize, however, that mental health is crucial for positive social and academic development. They are looking for an efficient way to invest in mental health that makes sense for their children and the school community more broadly.

Where should they begin this decision process? A good place to start would be to define their objectives. In other words, they need to specify which outcomes, precisely, they wish to improve. Mental health and related terms such as "social and emotional well-being" are concepts that can be defined in different ways. They need to choose their primary outcomes intentionally and thoughtfully. Next, the school's decision makers will need to examine their constraints. What amounts of resources—including money, class time, staff time, and expertise—could realistically be dedicated to this initiative? They also need to account for support or resistance from parents and other stakeholders, and how those factors might be leveraged or countered.

The school leaders can now begin to select an investment strategy that fits their objectives and constraints. Presumably, they will want to focus on strategies that have evidence of being effective in achieving their desired outcomes. In reviewing their options, they will need to figure out which evidence to look at, how to make

Investing in Children's Mental Health. Daniel Eisenberg and Ramesh Raghavan, Oxford University Press.
© Oxford University Press 2024. DOI: 10.1093/oso/9780190942014.003.0002

sense of that evidence, and how to translate the evidence into their setting and context. In many cases the investment strategy will be the implementation of a particular program, or set of programs, but it might also be new or revised practices and policies. Once they have settled on *what* they want to implement, their work has only just begun, as now they will also need to determine *how* to implement their chosen strategy in a way that maximizes its success and long-term sustainability.

Considering this challenging set of steps, it would not be surprising if many schools never make it through this decision-making and implementation process, if they even manage to get started. The process is similarly daunting in other contexts related to children's and youth mental health, such as home visiting for families with infants, the juvenile justice system for adolescents, and everything in between; the same types of considerations and challenges are relevant for every age group within childhood and adolescence and every level of public policy and organizational decision-making. This book aims to encourage and inform this process of deliberate, evidence-driven decision-making. While the challenges are steep, the health and well-being of children are too important to ignore.

Defining Children's Mental Health

Different ways of defining mental health can lead to very different investment priorities. For example, a definition that focuses on the severe end of the continuum of mental health, such as acute crises and the most impairing clinical disorders, might favor strategies that increase access to specialized mental health services for the relatively small percentage of children with the most urgent needs. In contrast, a definition that emphasizes emotional wellness and resilience would give more weight to universal prevention or health promotion strategies. For the purpose of identifying best investments, we prefer broad, holistic definitions of mental health, such as that described by the World Health Organization (2005): *Child and adolescent mental health is the "... capacity to achieve and maintain optimal psychological functioning and wellbeing."* This definition acknowledges the wide range of potential opportunities to improve young people's well-being through their mental health through not only treatment but also prevention and promotion.

Settling on a concept and measure of children's mental health is made more difficult by the fact that the United States does not have a consistent and complete mental health surveillance system. There is no systematic effort to track the state of mental health among children—or any other age group for that matter—across communities nationwide. There are also a wide variety of measures and methods, which lead to highly varying estimates of the prevalence of mental health conditions (Perou et al., 2013). This lack of standardization in measurement adds challenges in comparing priorities and tracking progress. Nevertheless, a community such as the school in our example has many reasonable options. Once they settle on the specific goals or objectives they wish to pursue, they should be able to find suitable measures to track progress.

Defining Best Investments

Best investments can also be defined in many different ways. There is, however, a set of standard practices in economic evaluation that we can apply to our context. These practices include tools such as benefit–cost analysis, cost-effectiveness analysis, and return-on-investment analysis, all of which share the same general purpose: to quantify the total benefits that can be derived from a limited set of resources. These tools are based on a utilitarian philosophy of social welfare, in which the objective is to maximize the total social benefit of policies and programs.

Among the different versions of economic evaluation, one of the main distinctions is between cost-effectiveness analysis, which calculates the economic cost required to achieve health gains, versus benefit–cost and return-on-investment analyses, which translate not only costs but also benefits into financial terms (i.e., dollars in the U.S. context). Cost-effectiveness analysis tends to be more popular in medicine and public health, where there is a reluctance to translate health into dollar values, whereas benefit–cost and return-on-investment analyses are common in the fields of education, juvenile justice, and child development more broadly.

Approaches to economic evaluation can also differ significantly in the perspectives they take. A narrower perspective limits its focus to the benefits and costs for a particular organization or payer, such as a school, community, insurance program, or the government. A broader perspective, the "societal perspective," considers all benefits and costs affected by an investment decision, regardless of who is responsible for paying or who benefits. Analyses can also differ in their time horizon, which has important implications for investments that target young people with the hope of improving their lifetime outcomes. In most situations it is useful to examine results from multiple perspectives; the long-run, societal perspective represents the idealistic, holistic view, whereas the short-run, organizational or public budget perspective acknowledges the reality that many decision makers have incentives to produce favorable outcomes, or at least balance their budgets, within a short time frame.

Another important caveat for economic evaluation tools is that they focus on overall well-being for a community, which is different from focusing on inequities in the distribution of well-being. Some version of economic evaluation, such as distributional cost-effectiveness analysis (Asaria et al., 2016), account for equity considerations, but these methods are rarely used in practice. Standard economic evaluation tools are particularly useful when addressing which strategy to take for a specific community or population rather than a broader question about which population or community to prioritize. In fact, there is an opportunity for economic analysis to help reduce inequities by identifying the most efficient strategies by which to improve outcomes within communities or populations that have been disadvantaged. As we will see later in this book, some of the programs with the strongest economic evidence are designed to support families and children with the greatest needs.

As this discussion is revealing, there are important nuances and limitations to economic analyses, which means they should be interpreted with some caution. These challenges are compounded by issues specific to the context of children's mental health. It can be difficult to measure mental health and behavioral outcomes for children and to translate the value of those outcomes into economic terms that can be compared with other priorities such as academic progress and achievement. In addition, there are major gaps in the evidence base upon which economic estimates depend; in particular, there is a lack of rigorous causal evidence for the effectiveness of many potential investments in children's mental health, particularly for longer-run outcomes (National Research Council, 2014).

Despite these caveats, our stance is that economic evidence such as benefit–cost analysis should be used as a major input into investment decisions for children's mental health. Economic evaluation provides a standardized, objective, quantitative framework through which to incorporate all available data and evidence. The perfect should not get in the way of the good. If we wait until every caveat is fully resolved, we will never use any rigorous method for quantifying the appeal of alternative options. It is better to make use of the available data to the extent possible, and to be knowledgeable and transparent about the accompanying limitations and assumptions.

Thus, we believe, the school leaders in our scenario should look at economic evidence regarding alternative investments they could make, to the extent such evidence is available. For example, if they look at school-based social-emotional learning (SEL) programs, they will find there are several programs with promising evidence of favorable benefit–cost ratios, even if this evidence is tentative in some respects. Thus, they might use the evidence to establish a preliminary list of alternatives, and then weigh that evidence alongside additional considerations such as parents' and communities' buy-in, their own capacity, and other issues related to implementation and sustainability.

Social-Ecological Framework

When selecting optimal investment strategies for its community, the school would ideally have a clear theory or logic about how potential investments would affect their children's well-being and mental health. This theory or logic would clarify the processes or pathways by which the programs under consideration would lead to better mental health outcomes. Mental health influences, and is influenced by, nearly every imaginable aspect of children's lives and therefore can only be properly examined through a broad, multilayered framework. This calls for a social-ecological framework, which acknowledges the many nested layers of influence around young people's lives (Emmons, 2000).

These factors range from internal (e.g., cognitive development and resilience skills such as self-soothing), to interpersonal (e.g., friendships, relationships with parents and teachers), to factors at the class and school level (e.g., resources, attitudes, expectations), to community-level and societal-level factors (e.g., public policies and programs, neighborhood safety, economic inequality, and corporate marketing). Each level of influence points to a set of potential risk and protective factors, with accompanying intervention strategies. For example, the interpersonal and social dynamics within a classroom are important for establishing norms, attitudes, and expectations, and these factors then give rise to intervention strategies such as SEL programs that foster cooperative, empathetic, and supportive relationships within that classroom.

Levels of influence can interact with each other in this framework. For example, the Positive Action SEL program emphasizes internal processes, as embodied in its thoughts-feelings-actions framework, as well as interpersonal relationships, such as treating others the way you like to be treated (Flay & Allred, 2010). Children who are more skilled at the internal processes are in turn more able to engage in more positive interpersonal behaviors and develop mutually supportive relationships. Thus, intervention strategies often correspond to multiple levels within a social-ecological framework.

Our hypothetical school can draw on this broad framework by examining its own social ecology and thereby assess its greatest needs and opportunities. Its social ecology would likely include strengths and deficits not only at the individual student level, but also in students' peer relationships, student–teacher relationships, family–teacher relationships, classroom dynamics, and out-of-class behaviors and opportunities (e.g., lunch, recess), all of which are embedded within a community ecology that includes social services, parks, neighborhoods, and more. The school can examine these levels to identify opportunities and challenges that might be addressed or leveraged with alternative investments and focus their attention on intervention strategies accordingly. A careful examination of its social ecology can also help illuminate opportunities to improve equity in a school community. For example, play is an important and necessary activity of childhood, one associated with many social, physical, and emotional benefits. However, some students in some schools may live in environments where playing outdoors is unsafe. In such communities, school leaders might expand after-school access to school facilities and implement other measures to keep children safe while they play within the school environment.

Developmental Perspective

While the social-ecological perspective more or less represents the space continuum surrounding children's mental health, the developmental perspective represents the time continuum. The needs and capacities of young people change over time, often dramatically so, with the result that they might respond best to very different intervention strategies at different stages of development (Masten & Barnes, 2018). The process of growing and maturing also brings new challenges and expectations, such as substance use and other risky behaviors that emerge in adolescence.

An organization or community, such as our hypothetical elementary school, may contain children across a wide range of developmental stages. Kindergarteners are typically five- or six-year-olds learning basic skills such as reading and developing friendships, whereas fifth graders are 10-to-11-year-olds learning about fractions, advanced grammar, and new social and behavioral challenges that emerge during puberty and early adolescence. Thus, the elementary school will need to consider how alternative investment strategies account for the changing needs of their children as they develop. Some intervention packages already account for this and are designed for a wide age range, with skills building upon each other from one grade to the next ("scaffolding" is the term often used in education). The school may also want to consider implementing different programs at different grade levels.

Nurturing Environments

The nurturing environments framework proposed by Biglan and colleagues (2012) offers another useful lens through which to consider strategies for investing in children's mental health. This framework advocates for a more unified approach to child wellbeing. It draws a deliberate contrast with current strategies that tend to focus on problems one by one, as reflected in separate programs and agencies focused on mood disorders, suicide risk, substance use, juvenile delinquency, special education, and so on. In this framework, a nurturing environment is the common thread in all strategies to improve children's mental health and well-being. Such environments have four key characteristics, according to the framework: first, they minimize biologically and psychologically toxic events and exposures; second, they teach, promote, and richly reinforce prosocial behavior, including self-regulatory behaviors; third, they monitor and limit opportunities for problem behavior; and fourth, they foster psychological flexibility—the ability to be mindful of one's thoughts and feelings and act in the service of one's values. This framework offers a compelling set of principles that could be promoted in a national and international public health campaign. As we will see in the case studies in later chapters, many of the most successful programs to address children's mental health are very consistent with the principles of a nurturing environment.

Integrating These Frameworks

The frameworks in this chapter are enmeshed in all subsequent chapters in the book, as we summarize best investments, investigate case studies, and distill themes and conclusions. A holistic definition of mental health, in combination with the basic principles of economic evaluation, forms the basis for how we define best investments. The social-ecological, developmental, and nurturing environments frameworks provide maps for how alternative interventions can generate positive outcomes, how they relate to each other, and how they might fit together in combinations within communities and society more broadly. Mental health as influenced by these social-ecological and developmental frameworks also informs our definition of child well-being (Raghavan & Alexandrova, 2015), which we will discuss as a key outcome in a later chapter. As illustrated in the case studies, these frameworks are essential for understanding the successes of programs to date and opportunities for progress toward even better investments in children's mental health in the future.

References

Asaria, M., Griffin, S., & Cookson, R. (2016). Distributional cost-effectiveness analysis: A tutorial. *Medical Decision Making, 36*(1), 8–19.

Biglan, A., Flay, B. R., Embry, D. D., & Sandler, I. N. (2012). The critical role of nurturing environments for promoting human well-being. *American Psychologist, 67*(4), 257–271.

Emmons, K. M. (2000). Health behaviors in a social context. In L. F. Berkman & I. Kawachi (Eds.), *Social Epidemiology* (pp. 242–265). Oxford University Press.

Flay, B. R., & Allred, C. G. (2010). The positive action program: Improving academics, behavior, and character by teaching comprehensive skills for successful learning and living. In T. Lovat, R. Toomey, & N. Clement (Eds.), *International research handbook on values education and student wellbeing* (pp. 471–501). Springer.

Masten, A. S., & Barnes, A. J. (2018). Resilience in children: Developmental perspectives. *Children, 5*(7), Article 98. https://www.mdpi.com/2227-9067/5/7/98

National Research Council. (2014). *Considerations in applying benefit-cost analysis to preventive interventions for children, youth, and families: Workshop summary.* National Academies Press.

Perou, R., Bitsko, R. H., Blumberg, S. J., Pastor, P., Ghandour, R. M., Gfroerer, J. C., & Huang, L. (2013). Mental health surveillance among children—United States, 2005–2011. *MMWR Supplements, 62*(2), 1–35.

Raghavan, R., & Alexandrova, A. (2015). Toward a theory of child well-being. *Social Indicators Research, 121*, 887–902.

World Health Organization. (2005). *Child and adolescent mental health policies and plans.* World Health Organization. Retrieved July 4, 2023, from https://apps.who.int/iris/handle/10665/43068

2

Overview of Current Evidence and Practice

Why Rely on Evidence?

A central assumption in this book is that *evidence* is the starting point for identifying and making the best investments in children's mental health. This assumption is important to question before we assess current evidence and practice.

Why should evidence be the first place we look for best investments? In the simplest terms, evidence gives us confidence that a program or service will achieve its intended outcomes. Evidence is typically collected through research and program evaluations and reflects the experiences of both providers and consumers of interventions and services. The information contained in evidence also should reflect the local context, recognizing that much of evidence is place and time based (Rycroft-Malone et al., 2004). Evidence assures a consumer, practitioner, or decision maker that an intervention actually does what it is designed to do. If you buy a car, television, or other expensive product, you want to be confident that it will work. Considering the stakes, we should hold investments in children's mental health to the same standard.

In the absence of clear evidence, there is plenty of reason to be skeptical as to whether any particular health or social intervention works. Across a range of fields, including education, medicine, job training, and business, most interventions are eventually determined to have weak or no benefits, even when they start with promising results (Coalition for Evidence-Based Policy, 2019).

Investing in Children's Mental Health. Daniel Eisenberg and Ramesh Raghavan, Oxford University Press.
© Oxford University Press 2024. DOI: 10.1093/oso/9780190942014.003.0003

Even programs with positive results from an initial RCT, the gold standard of evidence, often turn out to be ineffective in subsequent studies (Arnold Ventures, 2017; Ioannidis, 2005). A classic book on public policy by James Scott details the many reasons why government programs do not work as intended (Scott, 1999). For example, programs are often not implemented in the ideal way in which they were initially tested, or they might not be suited to all of the local contexts in which they are implemented.

The challenges in developing and delivering effective programs highlights the importance of a careful, discriminating approach to evidence. We need to focus much of our limited resources on the select programs that have been repeatedly shown to work in various settings and with differing populations. Such interventions are said to be *generalizable,* and one can reasonably have confidence that they will work in a novel setting.

Our investment strategies also need to expand the amount and quality of evidence. Along with investing heavily in implementing proven programs, there should also be significant investment in experimentation with new programs, accompanied by rigorous evaluation to document and learn about their effectiveness. Rigorous evaluation typically means large studies with a randomized control or other credible study design, and ideally some of the evidence is generated by independent evaluators with no stake in the outcomes.

There has been some general movement toward evidence-based policymaking in the United States in recent decades (Baron, 2018), and this movement has occurred not only at the federal level but also at the state and local level in many parts of the country (Pew-MacArthur Results First Initiative, 2018), with notable examples such as New Mexico and Minnesota (Pew-MacArthur Results First Initiative, 2019). Overall, this movement has been more robust in medicine and public health, where outcomes have greatly improved in many areas, and less so for social and behavioral programs and services, where many key outcomes have stagnated for decades (Arnold Ventures, 2019). As

Jon Baron, founder of the Coalition for Evidence-Based Policy, discusses, ". . . evidence-based approaches have so far gained only a foothold in social policy; the majority of social spending is still allocated with little regard to rigorous evidence about what works" (Baron, 2018).

It is important to note that we are only talking here about research evidence, and research evidence is but one leg of the traditional "three-legged stool" of evidence-based medicine (Sackett et al., 1996). Clinician judgment and expertise, and client voice— the other two legs—should also play a role in determining what interventions to deploy. After all, no one would want a scenario where policymakers force the delivery of a well-studied intervention that feels inappropriate or unhelpful to practitioners or participants themselves; such a scenario is unlikely to lead to good outcomes.

So, clearly nuance is important. But the primary focus, we argue, should be on research evidence. Research evidence should be one of the first considerations when determining the best course of action. Increasing the role of evidence in policy investments will allow us to escape from a Catch-22 cycle: We know the evidence base has flaws and gaps, so we avoid relying too much on evidence, which in turn weakens the incentive to produce and communicate good evidence. Without strong research evidence, we are often stuck in a situation where we rely only weakly on evidence to guide decisions about social programs, or we relax our standards for what constitutes good evidence in order to justify investments. Imagine the positive version of this cycle: If we truly rely on rigorous evidence to guide investment decisions, we could focus our investments on the small number of programs with such evidence, and, by necessity, we would redouble our efforts to produce that level of evidence for additional programs.

Classifying and Grading Evidence

Once we agree that evidence should be an important input into decision-making about investing in children's mental health, we need to consider how to summarize and interpret evidence effectively. Evidence is inevitably complex, resulting from many studies with a variety of strengths and limitations. Typically, the evidence for any given program or service gets boiled down to something like the following three categories: *excellent or strong evidence*, where there is high confidence that the program has positive effects; *promising evidence*, where there is favorable evidence that is nevertheless incomplete or mixed; and *poor or weak evidence*, where there is little or no evidence that the positive effects outweigh any negative effects. Sometimes it is important to divide this latter category further into programs with *incomplete* evidence versus those with clear evidence of being *ineffective*; the former group of programs require additional evaluation and research, whereas the latter group should be discontinued or modified substantially. The categories above map to the U.S. Preventive Services Task Force's well-known letter grading for evidence: roughly, a grade of A represents excellent evidence, B represents good or promising evidence, C represents mixed evidence, D represents poor evidence, and I represents incomplete evidence.

While it is useful to divide programs into discrete levels of evidence, the reality is of course more complicated. Within each rating level some programs might have significantly stronger evidence than others, and frequently a program has stronger evidence on some dimensions but weaker evidence on other dimensions. These nuances are important to consider in cases where a single program does not emerge from a review of evidence as the obvious winner for a community's needs and objectives.

Types of Evidence

When assessing the quality of evidence for a program or service, it is useful to distinguish between *internal* and *external* validity of evidence. In short, internal validity means that the estimated effectiveness is accurate for the specific context—such as a particular community or demographic group—for which the evaluation was conducted. External validity means that the estimate is relevant to broader contexts. It usually makes sense to think first about internal validity and then about external validity, when appraising evidence. If the evidence has high internal validity, then it is meaningful at least for the context in which it was produced and perhaps other similar contexts. If the evidence has low internal validity due to a weak research design, then external validity becomes moot, because we cannot trust the results even for the specific setting in which the program was tested.

If evidence comes from a well-conducted randomized trial, we can typically be confident of the program's internal validity, at least for the average participant in that trial. If evidence is from a nonrandomized comparison of groups, we need to consider carefully the selection process: Who or what factors determined who received the intervention (and which providers or organizations delivered it) versus the comparison condition; what does that imply about potential preexisting differences in the groups; and how well did the evaluation account for such differences?

External validity, on the other hand, is more speculative, because it is about whether and how we can generalize findings to other populations and settings. We can be more optimistic about external validity when an intervention has positive results in rigorous evaluations across diverse settings and populations. A challenge related to external validity is the projection of long-term outcomes, which are typically important for childhood interventions. Most commonly, long-term outcomes are projected through assumptions based on epidemiological data.

In the rare cases where long-term outcomes are directly observed in a study, as in the Perry Preschool Project (which involved a randomized trial in the early 1970s), for example, by the time we observe outcomes decades later in adulthood we need to ask how the context of the original intervention might translate to the current modern context.

Another important distinction is the *point estimate* for effectiveness versus the *uncertainty* surrounding that estimate. Policymakers and even researchers have a tendency to overemphasize the point estimate and underappreciate or understate the high amount of uncertainty surrounding much of the evidence that informs social policy decisions (Manski, 2013). The point estimate is typically viewed as the main result from an evaluation study; it refers to the specific number quantifying the effectiveness or cost-effectiveness of an intervention, such as a 20% reduction in depression symptoms or a 2.5 benefit–cost ratio. The uncertainty surrounding that estimate can be quantified by confidence intervals and p values. Typically, 95% confidence intervals are reported in evaluations; for example, the 20% reduction in depressive symptoms might have a 95% confidence interval ranging from 5% to 35%. In that case, an executive director considering the intervention for their agency can reasonably assume that the intervention will yield a beneficial effect (reducing depression), but the size of that beneficial effect will vary. At a societal level we need to find an appropriate balance between investing in programs with known effectiveness, alongside new programs with more potential upside and also more downside—uncertainty that could be reduced by conducting additional evaluations.

Next, an organization or community needs to consider not just the quality and types of evidence, as discussed thus far, but also the feasibility of implementing and sustaining a program or service. The effectiveness of an evidence-based intervention within an organization or community fundamentally depends on the fit between that intervention and the organization or community, and the capacity of that organization or community to deliver it appropriately. Social and behavioral programs are often complex to deliver, requiring substantial training, monitoring of fidelity and quality, and ongoing technical assistance. This represents an organizational challenge and upfront financial costs before the returns to that investment are realized. In addition to the initial costs, the ongoing costs of sustaining a program or service are often difficult to finance because the program or service might not fit neatly into existing funding schemes. Sometimes funding streams come to an end, and the agency is faced with the prospect of continuing an expensive program without any apparent source of support. The field of implementation science has begun to build a base of evidence for implementation strategies, typically involving technical assistance and support, to help overcome barriers, financial and otherwise, to the successful adoption and sustainment of evidence-based programs.

Lastly, an organization or community must balance the need for standardized evidence with the need to tailor investment decisions to their local culture and context. This relates to the previous point about external validity and generalizability. Taking this challenge one step further, evidence needs to be applied in a way that is sensitive to the differences across individuals within communities and organizations. For instance, an intervention that works for one cultural group may require significant adaptations before it is rolled out to another cultural group. While there are no easy answers to this challenge, one important path forward is to differentiate between core ingredients of effective interventions versus features that can be adapted and tailored without sacrificing effectiveness. We also need research studies that can quantify the level and focus of such adaptation. We revisit this and many of the other challenges described above throughout the remainder of this book.

"What Works" Registries

To help decision makers find and interpret the evidence on which programs are effective, a number of "what works" registries or clearinghouses have emerged in recent years. Among these registries, perhaps the best place to start when looking at programs affecting children's mental health is the Blueprints Programs for Healthy Youth Development (www.blueprintsprograms.org). Blueprints has two major advantages: It makes it easy to identify programs with the strongest evidence, and it includes a wide range of programs that are known to, or likely to, affect young people's mental health, cutting across many fields and sectors such as education, criminal justice, child development, and social work. Karl Hill, one of the principal investigators based at University of Colorado, told us that Blueprints views one of its key roles among registries as promoting high standards of evidence. For a program to be rated as a "Model" program, Blueprints requires multiple high-quality randomized trials with clear evidence of effectiveness extending beyond short-term outcomes. Hill notes that out of approximately 1,500 programs that have been assessed by Blueprints, only a small number (19 as of April 2023) have attained the Model designation, and only an additional 87 programs have been certified as Promising, the next tier of evidence. Thus, more than 90% of programs rated by Blueprints have not received any type of certification, either because their evidence is weak, incomplete, or both. Another benefit of Blueprints is that it emphasizes the feasibility of implementing programs; it only rates programs that provide clear guidance for implementing the program, and it provides information on how to obtain that guidance.

Communities looking to invest in effective programs for children's mental health should not necessarily limit their attention to Blueprints, which focuses mainly on community-based, preventive programs, and less so on clinical services. Considering the well-established gaps in the availability of mental health services for children, it is always worth examining whether increasing the supply of clinicians who can provide evidence-based services represents a strong investment. In addition, there are several other registries with relevant information for a range of programs related to children's mental health. Social Programs That Work (evidencebasedprograms.org) has high standards of evidence, much like Blueprints, and covers a variety of social, behavioral, and educational programs for all age groups. The Title IV-E Prevention Services Clearinghouse (https://prevent ionservices.acf.hhs.gov/) was established by the Administration for Children and Families (ACF) within the U.S. Department of Health and Human Services (HHS) to review programs and services that support children and families and prevent foster care placements. This Clearinghouse determines which programs are eligible for funding under the Families First welfare legislation— an example in which evidence plays a prominent and explicit role in policymaking. In addition, the CDC's Community Preventive Services Task Force (https://www.thecommunityguide.org/) offers summaries of evidence for various categories of programs. They have reviewed few programs to date related to children's mental health—only school-based cognitive behavioral therapy (CBT), for which they find strong evidence in favor of both universal and targeted delivery—but could be a useful resource to monitor in the coming years.

While much broader in scope than just children's mental health, the Cochrane Collaborative is another registry that can help inform decision-making in this area. A Cochrane Review is conducted by researchers who examine individual research studies, analyze their efficacy using a standardized approach in a systematic review, and then report them in a compendium called the Cochrane Library. The Cochrane Pregnancy and Childbirth group oversees reviews in the area of home visiting (pregnancy. cochrane.org), for example.

Each registry uses slightly different metrics of what constitutes an effective program (e.g., a randomized control trial along with two replications demonstrating that original effects held in different sites). Each also awards different labels for the best performing programs by their metric (Top Tier, and Near Top Tier, or Model Program and Promising Program, for example). For this reason, "evidence" is not a yes/no, bright line. It is a dimension, with programs having more or less evidence, based upon the number and strength of studies that go into the assessment of evidence.

The registry produced by the Washington State Institute for Public Policy (WSIPP) goes a step further than other registries by translating effectiveness into economic evidence, summarized as benefit–cost differentials and ratios. The WSIPP repository is also notable for the breadth of programs and services that it evaluates, spanning a range of social, educational, and health programs for all age groups, using a common framework for economic evaluation. The WSIPP estimates are also available in the Blueprints registry as supplemental information regarding economic evidence. One caveat for WSIPP's estimates is that they use data specific to Washington state, to the extent possible; their primary mission is to inform state-level policy decisions in Washington. We do not see this as a major drawback, however, because the main conclusions for economic evaluations of programs targeted to young people typically turn almost entirely on the main effect sizes for key outcomes such as education, health, and crime, which have large economic consequences in any context. In other words, the results for Washington state should be largely similar when extrapolated to other states and communities in the United States. In fact, the Pew-MacArthur Results First initiative has translated WSIPP's estimates to other states in their network. Perhaps a more important caveat is that WSIPP focuses on economic costs that can be readily quantified and does not attempt to assign monetary value to health and well-being per se, such as improvements in life expectancy and quality of life. This omission is understandable from the perspective of a state government's budget but can miss important benefits of programs and services focused on young people's mental health.

The growing number of registries has led to some confusion about which ones to use, particularly when the ratings are somewhat different from one registry to the next. To help users make sense of the various registries, the Results First initiative, first developed by the Pew Charitable Trusts and now maintained by Penn State University, offers a compendium of clearinghouses—in effect, a clearinghouse of clearinghouses—for programs related to social policy. Relatedly, a report by the Bridgespan Group provides a thorough review of clearinghouses and identifies opportunities for increasing their usefulness and impact (Neuhoff et al., 2015). For example, registries could be even more impactful if they provided easier access to contact information for peer organizations and communities that have successfully implemented a program or service, or if there were more active support and advice available to help decision makers use the registries effectively.

Looking across the evidence in the registries described above, we can make a few general observations. First, there is a relatively small number of programs with clear-cut evidence of being strong investments for children's mental health. Relatedly, there are a large number of programs that might or might not be strong investments as of now and require additional evidence. Next, the WSIPP is a valuable complement to other registries by providing economic evidence, and ideally there would also be a similar registry (or an expansion of the WSIPP registry) that takes a full societal perspective on measuring benefits and costs across the national context. Finally, these registries offer valuable information about what works but less guidance about how to implement and support these programs sustainably, although Blueprints and others do offer important information to help decision makers get started (Buckley et al., 2020).

Current Practice: Are We Making Good Investments?

Although the evidence base is far from perfect or complete, it highlights a small number of highly effective programs and services that could substantially improve mental health among children. But are we making those strong investments in the United States? Three sets of facts suggest that we are not making the best investments we could be making: alarming trends in distress and mental health among youth, lack of penetration of programs with the best evidence, and high penetration of some programs with poor or questionable evidence.

Perhaps the clearest evidence that we are not optimizing investments in children's mental health is simply the fact that mental health appears to be getting worse among young people in the United States. Depression, anxiety, suicide risk, and other indicators have risen substantially in recent years among adolescents and young adults (Twenge et al., 2019). The dramatic rise in social and digital media could help explain this recent rise (Twenge et al., 2018), but there were also steady declines in mental health in prior decades, which may have been related to more general changes to the social context affecting young people (Twenge et al., 2010). Regardless of the causes for the decline in mental health, it is clear that the available preventive and treatment programs and services have been inadequate on a population level. In addition, children and families have now been struggling with the COVID-19 pandemic for more than two years. The pandemic has caused severe economic strain for many families and has prevented children from attending school and other activities where they normally interact with friends, peers, and other supportive adults. Although the pandemic is a highly unusual event, it has further exposed the high levels of vulnerability for children's mental health in the United States and other countries.

A second concerning fact is that the programs with the best evidence of effectiveness and cost-effectiveness have generally achieved no more than modest penetration on a national level. In subsequent chapters we examine several examples of these programs, such as multisystemic therapy (MST), the Nurse–Family Partnership (NFP), and social-emotional learning (SEL) programs in schools such as Promoting Alternative Thinking Strategies (PATHS). In each case, the programs are estimated to reach no more than 5% of children and families who would likely benefit. Even in the example of school-based substance use prevention programs, where there has been considerable policy activity in recent decades, the most recent estimates indicate that fewer than one-fourth of schools are relying primarily on programs with strong evidence (Ringwalt et al., 2011).

The third point of concern is that many programs and services with weak evidence have achieved much higher penetration than those with strong evidence. As just noted, most schools use substance use prevention programs without good evidence of effectiveness. That example is highlighted by the long-standing dominance of the Drug Abuse Resistance Education (D.A.R.E.) program despite considerable evidence of ineffectiveness (West & O'Neal, 2004). Similarly, in the context of adolescents with severe behavioral problems, the most common approach has been to use punitive measures such as juvenile detention or other expensive residential programs with little evidence of effectiveness (Henggeler & Schoenwald, 2011).

The overall picture regarding current practice is far from ideal, and it is also far from complete. We need more systematic and precise data on the penetration of programs with varying levels of evidence. Relatedly, we need to monitor children's mental health more carefully at a population level in the United States, much like we have built surveillance systems for cancer and other health conditions, in order to identify opportunities for early intervention and prevention. In addition, we need to consider how current programs and services align not only with evidence of effectiveness but also with objectives to increase equity. In other words, do current intervention strategies prioritize communities and populations that are most disadvantaged with respect to the social and economic factors that exacerbate mental health risks? Do these programs and services adequately account for factors such as racism and other forms of discrimination that many children and families face, or do they account for factors such as food and housing insecurity? Currently, there is no systematic accounting of which programs and services are being delivered, whom they are reaching, and how this varies by socioeconomic and demographic group.

Why Are We Not Making Good Investments?

The main goal of this book is to make progress in understanding why as a society we are failing to make the best investments in children's mental health and how to improve the situation. The chapters that follow are focused on these challenges through a variety of case studies. Here we offer some general thoughts as a prelude to those discussions.

First, in some cases we do not fully understand the problem for which the evidence-based intervention is the solution. For example, an outdoor physical activity intervention to improve child health and well-being is likely to fail in communities where children are forbidden from playing outside the home because of the risk of neighborhood violence, and where an unspoken norm exists within the community that the local park is not meant for recreation. Perhaps an intervention emphasizing neighborhood safety is the more appropriate first step in this setting (Keener et al., 2009). The social determinants of mental health and emotional well-being need to be understood when identifying and implementing investment strategies.

Second, decision makers may not know what to do when confronted with a problem facing children within their community. Scientists refer to these as adoption decisions—which, out of a possible universe of interventions and solutions, can or should a decision maker choose to adopt? Providing this type of decision support is the purpose of registries like those discussed earlier in this chapter. Another strategy is to foster meaningful relationships between researchers, community-based stakeholders, and decision makers. Community-participatory partnered research promotes these relationships (Jones & Wells, 2007). Much of the onus here lies on the research community, which needs to better bridge the gap between what is interesting for science, and what is necessary for population well-being.

Third, even when we have identified a problem and possess a solution, we may not know how to deliver an intervention for a new population and context. The key challenge is to ensure that the elements that make the intervention effective are preserved, even as the intervention is changed in ways that enhance its generalizability. In Chapter 8, we will return to this topic of intervention design and implementation. An entire field of research, implementation science, has rapidly developed during the past four decades in response to the well-known gap between what we ought to do, and what we actually end up doing. Consequently, we have the benefit of a great deal of scholarship that can help guide these efforts in the context of children's mental health.

Implementation science and related research have highlighted several other factors that are important for understanding the challenge of disseminating and sustaining effective practices. Given the resource constraints under which many mental health agencies operate, ensuring organizational capacity for implementation is crucial (Aarons et al., 2018). Building this capacity involves working with leadership and providers to assure commitment and ensuring that the organization has systems and processes in place to absorb, deliver, and monitor the intervention. In some cases, it may be necessary to stop delivering older or less effective programs and services to free up resources for new ones; this process is called "deimplementation" (van Bodegom-Vos et al., 2017). Organizations must be able to afford implementation efforts, and financial incentives at varying levels of the implementation ecology must be aligned correctly in order to sustain services and programs (Raghavan et al., 2008). More recently, the critical role of purveyor organizations has received long overdue attention. These organizations, also referred to as intermediary/purveyor organizations (IPOs), have an explicit objective to facilitate the dissemination, implementation, and sustainability of programs and services. Over 90% of evidence-based interventions (EBIs) for children's mental health in the Substance Abuse and Mental Health Services Administration's (SAMHSA's) National Registry of Evidence-Based Programs and Practices (NREPP; now known as the Evidence-Based Practices Resource Center) have one or more IPO facilitating dissemination and implementation, according to a review by Proctor and colleagues (2019). Most of these IPOs engaged in many different implementation strategies within the broader domains of education/training, planning, financing, quality management, and restructuring. Education and training were the most common types of strategy. The review noted that we need more research on which strategies are most effective or whether it is simply necessary to use a large number of different strategies. Another recent review by the Bridgespan group provides additional insight into the strengths and limitations of purveyor organizations supporting social and health programs for children and youth, highlighting that many purveyors lack the financial incentives and entrepreneurial skills to expand the reach of programs (Neuhoff et al., 2017).

Summary and Conclusion

In this chapter we have argued that evidence is the starting point for best investments. We discussed key considerations when making sense of evidence and examined the current state of evidence for programs affecting children's mental health. That evidence is modest relative to what we would ideally like to know but still offers crucial guidance about a small number of programs that are strong investments. It is painfully clear, however, that as a society we are not consistently making these best investments. In the chapters that follow, we examine specific cases of programs and services that illustrate both the potential and the challenges in making better investments. The purpose of these case studies is to add texture to these issues and gain new clues regarding how to improve investments in children's mental health.

References

Aarons, G. A., Moullin, J. C., & Ehrhart, M. G. (2017). The role of organizational processes in dissemination and implementation research. In R. C. Brownson, G. A. Colditz, & E. K. Proctor (Eds.), *Dissemination and implementation research in health: Translating science to practice* (pp. 121–142). Oxford University Press.

Arnold Ventures. (2017). *If at first you succeed, try again!* (Straight Talk on Evidence). https://www.straighttalkonevidence.org/2017/08/16/if-at-first-you-succeed-try-again/

Arnold Ventures. (2019). *FDR's call for "bold, persistent experimentation": An antidote to 40-year stagnation in key areas of social policy.* https://www.straighttalkonevidence.org/2019/01/11/fdrs-call-for-bold-persistent-experimentation-an-antidote-to-40-year-stagnation-in-key-areas-of-social-policy-part-two-in-a-series/

Baron, J. (2018). A brief history of evidence-based policy. *The ANNALS of the American Academy of Political and Social Science, 678*(1), 40–50.

Buckley, P. R., Fagan, A. A., Pampel, F. C., & Hill, K. G. (2020). Making evidence-based interventions relevant for users: A comparison of requirements for dissemination readiness across program registries. *Evaluation Review, 44*(1), 51–83.

Coalition for Evidence-Based Policy. (2019). *Practical evaluation strategies for building a body of proven-effective social programs.* https://craftmediabuc ket.s3.amazonaws.com/uploads/Practical-Evaluation-Strategies-updated-Mar-2019.pdf

Henggeler, S. W., & Schoenwald, S. K. (2011). Evidence-based interventions for juvenile offenders and juvenile justice policies that support them and commentaries. *Social Policy Report, 25*(1), 1–28.

Ioannidis, J. P. (2005). Why most published research findings are false. *PLoS Medicine, 2*(8), Article e124.

Jones, L., & Wells, K. (2007). Strategies for academic and clinician engagement in community-participatory partnered research. *Journal of the American Medical Association, 297*(4), 407–410.

Keener, D., Goodman, K., Khan, L. K., Lowry, A., & Zaro, S. (2009). *Recommended community strategies and measurements to prevent obesity in the United States: Implementation and measurement guide.* CDC.

Manski, C. F. (2013). *Public policy in an uncertain world: Analysis and decisions.* Harvard University Press.

Neuhoff, A., Axworthy, S., Glazer, S., & Berfond, D. (2015). *The what works marketplace: Helping leaders use evidence to make smarter choices.* Bridgespan Group. https://www.bridgespan.org/bridgespan/Images/artic les/the-what-works-marketplace/the-what-works-marketplace.pdf

Neuhoff, A., Loomis, E., & Ahmed, F. (2017). *What's standing in the way of the spread of evidence-based programs.* Bridgespan Group.

Pew-MacArthur Results First Initiative. (2018). *How counties can use evidence-based policymaking to achieve better outcomes.* https://www.pewtrusts.org/ en/research-and-analysis/reports/2018/12/10/how-counties-can-use-evidence-based-policymaking-to-achieve-better-outcomes

Pew-MacArthur Results First Initiative. (2019). *Minnesota and New Mexico demonstrate the power of evidence in policymaking.* https://www.pewtrusts. org/en/research-and-analysis/issue-briefs/2019/11/minnesota-and-new-mexico-demonstrate-the-power-of-evidence-in-policymaking

Proctor, E., Hooley, C., Morse, A., McCrary, S., Kim, H., & Kohl, P. L. (2019). Intermediary/purveyor organizations for evidence-based interventions in the US child mental health: characteristics and implementation strategies. *Implementation Science, 14*(3), 1–14.

Raghavan, R., Bright, C. L., & Shadoin, A. L. (2008). Toward a policy ecology of implementation of evidence-based practices in public mental health settings. *Implementation Science, 3*(1), 1–9.

Ringwalt, C., Vincus, A. A., Hanley, S., Ennett, S. T., Bowling, J. M., & Haws, S. (2011). The prevalence of evidence-based drug use prevention curricula in U.S. middle schools in 2008. *Prevention Science, 12*(1), 63–69.

Rycroft-Malone, J., Seers, K., Titchen, A., Harvey, G., Kitson, A., & McCormack, B. (2004). What counts as evidence in evidence-based practice? *Journal of Advanced Nursing, 47*(1), 81–90.

Sackett, D., Rosenberg, W., Muir-Gray, J., Haynes, R., & Richardson, W. (1996). Evidence-based medicine: What it is and what it isn't. *British Medical Journal, 312,* 71–72.

Scott, J. (1999). *Seeing like a state: How certain schemes to improve the human condition have failed.* Yale University Press.

Twenge, J. M., Cooper, A. B., Joiner, T. E., Duffy, M. E., & Binau, S. G. (2019). Age, period, and cohort trends in mood disorder indicators and suicide-related outcomes in a nationally representative dataset, 2005–2017. *Journal of Abnormal Psychology, 128*(3), 185–199.

Twenge, J. M., Gentile, B., DeWall, C. N., Ma, D., Lacefield, K., & Schurtz, D. R. (2010). Birth cohort increases in psychopathology among young Americans, 1938–2007: A cross-temporal meta-analysis of the MMPI. *Clinical Psychology Review, 30*(2), 145–154.

Twenge, J. M., Joiner, T. E., Rogers, M. L., & Martin, G. N. (2018). Increases in depressive symptoms, suicide-related outcomes, and suicide rates among US adolescents after 2010 and links to increased new media screen time. *Clinical Psychological Science, 6*(1), 3–17.

van Bodegom-Vos, L., Davidoff, F., & Marang-van de Mheen, P. J. (2017). Implementation and de-implementation: Two sides of the same coin? *BMJ Quality & Safety, 26*(6), 495–501.

West, S. L., & O'Neal, K. K. (2004). Project DARE outcome effectiveness revisited. *American Journal of Public Health, 94*(6), 1027–1029.

3

Home Visiting Programs

A few blocks over from Deidre's apartment lies the Robert F. Kennedy bridge where, on this crisp January morning, a row of cars resembles a metallic millipede inching its way toward Brooklyn. A high-pitched squeal rises from the carpeted living room. Deidre's 15-month-old, a boy named Dayvon, furrows his brow as he systematically dismantles a large, yellow plastic toy that may have been, at one point in its existence, a clock. Deidre turns to the other woman in the room, Liz, who is watching Dayvon with an indulgent smile.

"That's just a toy, but I have to keep a close eye on him—he keeps trying to rip out the duct tape," says Deidre with an amused shrug, pointing to a wall socket covered with blue-gray duct tape. Deidre has also secured with duct tape every single plug from floor lamps and other appliances inserted into wall sockets. Liz, who discussed child proofing on her last visit to Deidre's apartment two weeks ago, smiles and nods approval. Soon the two women are discussing strategies to get Dayvon to eat peas, since nutrition is an ongoing topic whenever Liz comes to visit.

Deidre lives in New York City, in the borough of the Bronx. In 2008, Heather Appel, a journalist writing for the *Daily News*, reported that pregnant women in Mott Haven, an area in the Bronx, have an infant mortality rate nearly twice that of the rest of New York City, and roughly the same as that of pregnant women in Uruguay (Appel, 2008). This is one of the problems for which Liz is the solution. Liz is a family support specialist, conducting home visits in some of New York City's most vulnerable neighborhoods.

Investing in Children's Mental Health. Daniel Eisenberg and Ramesh Raghavan, Oxford University Press.

Liz works for one of the several home visiting programs that offer services to women and their children in the state of New York (New York State Department of Health, 2019). There are two large home visiting programs operating in the state, along with several smaller programs. Nurse–Family Partnership (NFP), perhaps the best known and best supported home visiting program, enrolls first-time mothers who are less than 28 weeks pregnant. We will examine NFP later in this chapter. Another large program, Healthy Families New York, an affiliate of Healthy Families America, enrolls families who are pregnant or with a child less than three months old. The New York State Office of Children and Family Services (OCFS) funds three dozen Healthy Families New York programs in all five New York City boroughs, and in 24 counties statewide. Each year, around 5,600 families are visited by a Healthy Families family support specialist at an average cost of approximately $5,000 per family in New York City.

Home visiting is an umbrella term for programs in which a professional or a trained peer who is knowledgeable about parenting in early childhood visits parents and children in their homes (Sweet & Appelbaum, 2004). The professional can be a nurse, a community health worker, a social worker, or a specially trained program provider. The visits can either begin during pregnancy or shortly after childbirth, depending on the program. The home visitor can visit the home solo or accompanied by a peer. Once in the home, the visitor can focus on a range of topics and undertake a range of activities, all with the goal of supporting the health and well-being of the child and strengthening the parenting and family environment. The visitor can work with the child, the parent, or both (the "triadic" model). Typical areas that home visitors emphasize include providing information about child health and development, helping with meal preparation and nutrition, discussing the challenges of parenting, brokering infant healthcare services (e.g., immunizations and well-baby visits), leveraging various community resources needed by the family, providing legal referrals to persons with immigration-related challenges, and addressing the many other needs that a family might have in the immediate wake of childbirth. Some of these topics may be emphasized more in certain types of home visiting programs, and, as we shall see later on in the chapter, what is emphasized may change over time or with the changing needs of the family.

One subgroup of home visiting programs has a particular emphasis on infant mental health (Weatherston & Ribaudo, 2020). Infant mental health refers to the complete well-being of a developing child—interpersonal, cognitive, and emotional. Infants and toddlers do not just need to be fed and housed; they also need a caregiving environment within which they can develop and flourish (Lieberman, 2017). Home visiting programs, by focusing on particular outcomes such as the promotion of secure attachment between parents and children, improve infant and toddler mental health (Fraiberg, 1980). A successful example of these types of programs is Infant Mental Health–Home Visiting (Fraiberg, 1980); there are other approaches developed by other scholars with a similar emphasis (Weatherston & Ribaudo, 2020).

Nurse–Family Partnership

Home visiting is perhaps best thought of as a general approach with many "flavors" of differing intent, design, features, and intended outcomes. To illustrate, let us examine one well-studied home visiting program, NFP, in greater depth.

NFP aims to improve pregnancy outcomes, child development, and economic stability for at-risk families (Olds, 2006). While the program model has evolved somewhat since its origins, the core of the program involves nurses acting as home visitors to first-time mothers beginning during pregnancy and continuing through the child's second birthday. During 60-to-75-minute visits, which usually occur every other week, these nurses promote health-related behaviors during and after pregnancy, educate mothers about appropriate physical and emotional care of their infants, enhance links between parents and health and social support systems, and encourage the mother's personal development. The goal is to deliver around 64 visits in total, though the actual number of visits varies slightly depending on when during her pregnancy the client is enrolled in the program. NFP requires the first home visit to occur no later than the end of the woman's 28th week of pregnancy, though there is an adapted model where this criterion is relaxed. Another adaptation is for women who are pregnant with their second child. In 2020 alone, over 2,400 nurses delivered over 1.8 million NFP visits to over 58,000 families nationwide; after March 2020 almost all of these visits were delivered via videoconference or phone, as a result to the COVID pandemic (Nurse–Family Partnership, 2021).

The Home Visiting Evidence of Effectiveness (HomVEE) site is a compendium of early childhood home visiting programs (homvee.acf.hhs.gov), maintained by the U.S. Department of Health and Human Services, Administration for Children and Families. Written primarily for administrators and policymakers making decisions about home visiting programs to implement, the site summarizes research evaluations of NFP from 275 studies published since 1979. From the studies meeting HomVEE's quality standards, there is solid evidence that NFP improves outcomes for both children and mothers. For children these outcomes include lower rates of maltreatment and injuries and better indicators of health during infancy. The positive outcomes continue later in childhood (e.g., higher school readiness) and into adolescence; NFP children at age 15 were less likely to run away; had fewer arrests, convictions, and violations of probation; had fewer sex partners; drank less alcohol and smoked cigarettes less frequently; and were identified less often in child maltreatment reports (Miller, 2015). For mothers and families, positive outcomes for NFP include better maternal health, reductions in rapid repeat pregnancies, higher labor market participation, and lower dependence on public assistance programs.

Flexibility and Variation within and across Programs

A part of the Affordable Care Act in 2010, the Maternal, Infant, and Early Childhood Home Visiting (MIECHV) program considerably expanded home visiting services for vulnerable families. MIECHV funding supports home visiting programs that meet standards of evidence under HomVEE. Programs that have been most commonly supported under MIECHV are Early Head Start, Healthy Families America, NFP, and Parents as Teachers. These programs share an emphasis on a primary outcome—improving child health and development. However, Healthy Families America also focuses on child maltreatment prevention, NFP focuses on the health of the mother (in addition to the child), and Early Head Start and Parents as Teachers both emphasize positive parenting and school readiness. The programs also differ somewhat in their target population, with NFP focusing on first-time mothers, Healthy Families America focusing on families at risk for child maltreatment, and the other programs displaying broader eligibility criteria. While NFP is primarily a program that enrolls pregnant women, both Early Head Start and Parents as Teachers also enroll women with toddlers in the national evaluation. These programs also vary in terms of the provider delivering the program within the home. NFP employs professional nurses with at least a bachelor's degree, whereas the other programs are more flexible with respect to credentials: Early Head Start specifies domains of training and expertise in early childhood education among others, and Parents as Teachers and Healthy Families America both require program staff to have at least a high school education and relevant experience.

In addition to program emphasis, target populations, and provider qualifications, home visiting programs also differ in dose. NFP, as we have discussed earlier, targets a total of 64 visits, while most other programs have less intensive visit schedules. On the other hand, visit length also varies by program and is not always standardized within each program, so the dose of the program is highly variable across recipient families. Relatedly, while a home visitor has a protocol, this protocol is secondary to the needs of the particular family. The activities and lessons are delivered at various times and for various durations, and the protocol is rarely static in the face of crises that can arise suddenly in the lives of vulnerable families. The elements of a home visiting program are not fixed in the manner in which, say, the strength and frequency of taking a pill is fixed. It is almost as if the course of treatment consists of a set of pills, each specific to a particular health need, administered at varying doses and for varying durations, and supplemented by other treatments delivered by other providers.

Evidence of Effectiveness for Home Visiting Programs

Meta-analyses of home visiting programs, which sum up the effectiveness of programs across various studies, indicate that these programs generally demonstrate small but significant overall effects on the child's cognitive development, and parental behaviors and skills, among other outcomes (Filene et al., 2013). However, there is wide variability in the magnitude of these effects, the specific effect they produce (e.g., birth outcomes, or parenting skills improvement, child physical health, etc.), and in the particular elements of the program that produce these effects.

Another review examined effects from 21 studies of home visiting on specific outcomes for children of ages birth to six years old from disadvantaged families (Peacock et al., 2013). All of these studies had conducted randomized control trials (RCTs) to assess how effective home visiting was, most began services while the mother was pregnant, and most were conducted in the United States. The authors found that home visiting by paraprofessionals improved development and health outcomes for socially high-risk families with young children—these outcomes included child maltreatment prevention (when the program begins before childbirth), and improvements in cognitive development and reduced problem behaviors. Generally, effects were greater with greater numbers of visits. So, the timing and "dose" of these visits appear to be important. This emphasis on timing, content, and frequency—and the resultant effects—is perhaps one reason why NFP is considered a Model Program by Blueprints for Healthy Youth Development, the sole home visiting program to receive such a designation. It is also the sole Top Tier home visiting program, as evaluated by Social Programs That Work, although another home visiting program called Child FIRST has achieved Near Top Tier designation.

As part of the MIECHV program, a national evaluation study delivered four of the most popular home visiting programs to over 4,200 families across 12 states and compared them with controls using an RCT design. In 2019, the results of this evaluation were released (Michalopoulos et al., 2019). In contrast to the studies cited above, overall results in this evaluation were sobering. Out of a total of 12 "confirmatory" outcomes, statistically significant effects at the 15-month follow-up were observed for only 4; home visiting improved the quality of the home environment, enhanced parental supportiveness (i.e., reduced psychological aggression) toward the child, reduced the number of Medicaid-reimbursed emergency department visits, and reduced child behavior problems. None of these outcomes had consistently large effects—66 out of 67 different effects studied had an effect size smaller than 0.20 (an effect size smaller than 0.20 is typically considered a "small" effect), and the authors concluded that ". . . after adjusting for the number of confirmatory outcomes, none of the 12 estimated effects is statistically significant . . . this finding reduces the study team's confidence that any individual outcome was improved by the home visiting services that were studied" (p. ES-10).

The design of the study involved recipients of services from all four models being pooled together for purposes of analyses. The design did not compare effects of one program versus controls, or one program versus another. Hence, it is difficult to definitively answer the question of which programs work for which outcomes. Three out of four programs displayed identical effect sizes of 0.11 on improving the quality of the home environment; NFP had a smaller effect size of 0.05. On the other outcome of child emergency department visits, NFP was the standout model with an effect size of –0.5. Parents as Teachers had no effect on this outcome, while Early Head Start and Healthy Families America had smaller effects in the 0.2–0.3 range (an effect size of 0.5 is considered a "medium" effect.) These differences in the magnitude of effects are related to the foci of the program—NFP is a community health intervention delivered by nurses and is more medically focused than any of the other programs studied in the evaluation.

So, what should we make of such divergent answers to the question of whether home visiting works? The current scientific consensus seems to be that home visiting is certainly a promising way to serve families who may otherwise have difficulty in engaging in supportive services, and that home visiting has the potential for positive results among such families, particularly on healthcare usage and child development (Avellar & Supplee, 2013). Additionally, based on the national evaluation and other evidence, it appears that NFP has the firmest evidence base to date among the home visiting programs. We clearly have a long way to go before we fully understand which program components work to produce which outcomes, at what levels of intensity, for whom, and in what contexts.

Challenges in Establishing and
Preserving Effectiveness

Why is it difficult to establish clear evidence of effectiveness for most home visiting programs? The authors of the national evaluation offer several suggestions. First, the national evaluation was conducted at several sites across the country and may serve to average out effects observed in smaller, local evaluations. In other words, effects are not merely programmatic or internal; they are contextual or external. The same program delivered in identical ways in different places may produce different results. Second, prior efficacy studies cited were conducted on only one program, usually by the developers of the program, and the investigators of those studies "... might have chosen outcomes where those models were expected to make the largest differences" (p. ES-11). And the national evaluation results are not too different from the studies that we have cited earlier in this chapter that show some heterogeneity in the outcomes achieved by various home visiting programs.

Dr. Sue Stepleton, the former president and CEO of Parents as Teachers, shared with us some of her insights gained after nine years of running the national not-for-profit program. Home visiting programs are designed to be highly adaptable. While these characteristics allow greater tailoring of the program to the needs of families, they make the program less homogeneous. RCTs, the gold standard of scientific designs that establish how effective a program is, are best suited for programs that are fixed and unchangeable. If the actual "treatment" changes based on client need, randomized trials end up evaluating only portions of the treatment and consequently tend to show a lack of evidence. This is not a problem restricted to studies of home visiting—many studies of programs in the human services field show modest effectiveness because of the changeable nature of the program. Our ways of doing and our ways of knowing what is effective in what we are doing are somewhat misaligned.

Relatedly, most programs evolve over time as components are refined, as the team gains greater familiarity with the myriad problems they are attempting to solve, and as the client population and its needs change. Consequently, a particular home visiting program may look different in its, say, tenth year from that in its first year—in other words, it undergoes *adaptation*. This is not a major problem if one knows what the key program elements are that contribute to its effectiveness—then adaptation can proceed while preserving these key program elements and, thereby, assuring good client outcomes. Later on in this book, we discuss the idea of "core elements," also referred to as "core components" or "active ingredients." These specific program elements are key to the efficacy of the program and must not be tampered with if the program is to display its effects. Other aspects of the program can be modified or changed to make it better fit with the needs of the child and family without compromising effectiveness. Unfortunately, program developers and those who adapt the programs may not be always able to distinguish the core elements from the modifiable features and so can inadvertently "adapt away" some of what works. The more scientists identify the active components of home visiting programs, the easier it becomes to ensure their consistent effectiveness across the many flavors of home visiting programs.

Where a program has been implemented also matters—Parents as Teachers was implemented initially in well-funded school districts and was initially viewed as a program for middle-class, largely white families in Missouri. When programs migrate to another school district that is not as well resourced or has a different demographic profile, they can be replicated to some extent if there is adequate money that maintains the key program elements. However, state cutbacks in Missouri in 2009 resulted in poor implementation of Parents as Teachers in low-resource districts. In such circumstances, achieving the program's originally demonstrated outcomes becomes an unrealistic expectation.

A Population-Focused
Approach: Family Connects

Although most home visiting programs target families with particular risk factors such as poverty, this need not always be the case.
Dr. Benjamin Goodman, director of research and evaluation for a
nurse home visiting program called Family Connects in Durham,
North Carolina, spoke to us about the need for systems-level
approaches that engage families and connect them to resources and
services—including home visiting programs—based on identified
need. For Family Connects Durham, the need to demonstrate
population-level change led to the development of a model offered
to families of all children born in the county, essentially making it
a universal, countywide program (www.ccfhnc.org/programs/fam
ily-connects-durham/).

Family Connects Durham differs in another way from many
other home visiting programs—it is not offered to women before they give birth; instead, it is considered to be a part of post-
pregnancy health and social care. Women are identified through
hospitals and health facilities and are scheduled for between one
and three Family Connects Durham home visits. Given the scale of
the program, and the services that nurses need to be able to leverage
for their clients, it requires a range of high-quality community-
based resources. The program is effective, with two randomized
control trials demonstrating positive outcomes on maternal mental
health, fewer child protective services investigations for suspected
child maltreatment, and reduced emergency department use for
the child (Dodge et al., 2014, 2019). This success has come despite it
being a relatively brief program delivered after childbirth.

What, then, accounts for the success of Family Connects?
Dr. Goodman told us that, in his opinion, Family Connects is effective because it ". . . combines top-down identification and align-
ment of services and support for families with young children with
a bottom-up approach of engaging all families of newborns through

short-term nurse home visiting, identifying family-specific need, and connecting families with services and resources for long-term support." Family Connects is, by design, a *population* wellness program focused on improving population outcomes rather than individual outcomes. It is expressly designed for all children within a catchment area such as a county. Its positive effects, then, may be due to this population wellness emphasis, which is about not only delivering services to each family but also strengthening the community-level system of referrals and support. This thinking is aligned to programs that currently operate overseas using a similar universal model. In Sweden, for example, nurse home visiting is offered to all families nationwide regardless of income or risk status; families call a child health center (*barnavårdscentral*) to register their newborn, which triggers a nurse home visit. This is a public health approach—one that recognizes that one cannot treat one's way to population health, that determinants of well-being are contextual and not individual, and that different instruments and competencies are required when the outcomes are population focused than when an outcome is individual.

It is also likely that at least part of the reason for why Family Connects works so well is the location within which it is delivered— the observation that Dr. Stepleton also made in reference to the Missouri-based Parents as Teachers program. Durham lies in a region of the country that is anchored by three flagship universities, in the midst of one of the nation's largest knowledge, health, and innovation hubs. It is likely that this wealth of community and intellectual capital, in the midst of which this program is delivered, accounts for at least some of its early success. Today, Family Connects operates in 13 states, both in well-resourced sites (such as Long Island in New York) and comparatively less-resourced locations (such as Victoria County, Texas). As the program expands to less resource-intensive areas, it will need to continue to demonstrate positive effects in order to truly attain success as a population-level program.

The Economic Case for Home Visiting

Economic evaluations of home visiting are largely positive. Home visiting programs have been subject to a series of economic evaluations; the first trial of NFP in Elmira, New York, revealed that, among a sample of 400 women, public spending was less than the costs of the program for low-income mothers (Olds et al., 1993). The study took into account expenditures on Aid to Families with Dependent Children (AFDC), food stamps, Medicaid, and child protective services, and it subtracted from this amount tax revenues from mothers' employment. By the time the children were four years of age, government savings per family amounted to $1,772 for the sample as a whole and $3,498 for low-income families. Subsequent economic evaluations have also reported that NFP reduces the prevalence of several adverse outcomes such as preterm births, maltreatment incidents, youth substance use, and child injuries; these outcomes could potentially avert the need for approximately 4.8 million months of child Medicaid spending nationally. Overall safety net spending—Medicaid, Temporary Assistance for Needy Families (TANF), and Supplemental Nutrition Assistance Program (SNAP) food benefits—may reduce by approximately $3 billion (Miller, 2015). Given that NFP would cost approximately $1.6 billion to implement nationally, this reflects a sound return on investment. Benefit–cost ratios for NFP range between 1.3 and 6.5 (societal perspective) and between 0.2 and 5.0 (government perspective), generally suggesting strong rates of return (Miller, 2013).

A particularly attractive aspect of NFP is its emphasis on low-income families, and the fact that its economic returns are greatest for these highly vulnerable families. Miller estimates that state and federal governments recover between 2.2 and 8.2 times the amount of money that they spend on services for these vulnerable children (Miller, 2013). Reduced spending on Medicaid accounts for the greatest returns—NFP reduces Medicaid spending by 12% for the first-born child beneficiary, yielding approximately $20,000 in savings per family served. This is not surprising given that NFP is the most medically focused home visiting program that we have reviewed, and that healthcare costs are extraordinarily high in the United States when compared with those of other developed economies. Overall savings—accounting for reductions in special education, child maltreatment, and criminal justice costs—approach $37,000 per family. Other studies have used the quality-adjusted life year (QALY) as a metric. Using this metric, studies examining low-income families report that deployment of NFP would generate 0.2 QALYs per child, with a net benefit of $2,764 per child (Wu et al., 2017).

On average, NFP, the most expensive home visiting program in a recent analysis, costs $7,596 per family; these costs are largely driven by staff salaries, since the program requires bachelor's-level nurses to provide all services. Parents as Teachers, the least expensive program, costs $2,415 per family (Burwick et al., 2014). Given that many of these programs are multi-month or multi-year programs delivering care to clients with diverse needs, another way to look at costs is to examine per-visit costs. These costs range from an average of $210 per visit (Parents as Teachers) to $673 (Healthy Families America). Given the magnitude of returns that these costs provide, home visiting appears to represent a worthwhile investment of public funds, although there are still questions about the consistency of impacts, as discussed earlier.

Equity Considerations

Equity considerations have been a key design element of home visiting programs since their inception. NFP was developed primarily to serve socioeconomically disadvantaged mothers. As a model, NFP has displayed generally positive findings in RCTs across three different settings with very different low-income populations—Elmira, New York (400 mostly white families in a rural area), Memphis, Tennessee (1,138 mostly African American families in an urban area), and Denver, Colorado (735 mostly Latinx families in areas of mixed urbanicity). As we have reviewed above, the effects of NFP are pronounced on safety net spending—Medicaid, TANF, and SNAP food benefits—helping to reduce families' reliance on these important programs for people experiencing poverty.

Home visiting programs have adapted their service models that have an explicit equity focus (Lewy, 2021). Home visiting programs such as NFP train their staff in antiracism and implicit bias, and several programs train staff in delivering culturally appropriate care. Home visiting has also been adapted to make the model more culturally relevant; for example, Family Spirit is a model designed specifically for American Indian families that demonstrated increased knowledge of, and involvement in, child rearing in an RCT conducted in one Apache and three Navajo territories (Barlow et al., 2006). Finally, home visiting programs are designed to increase service access—narrative reviews of programs have found positive effects on immunization completion, asthma control, well-child visits, and other healthcare-related services (Williams et al., 2008). Through such effects on increasing appropriate utilization of services, particularly for the low-income families that they serve, home visiting programs may reduce health disparities among the most vulnerable of the nation's children. It will be important for home visiting programs to continue to build on their important role in promoting a more equitable society.

Conclusion

Home visiting programs have many beneficial effects for child and family outcomes. These benefits are achieved at relatively modest costs, and even the most expensive home visiting programs display a positive return on investment. It is true that we need to know more about what program characteristics are associated with the greatest returns on investments, and for whom. Future research will need to resolve some of the uncertainties and contradictory findings that we have highlighted in this chapter. Nevertheless, in the light of the current state of knowledge, home visiting programs represent worthy targets for public investments, particularly programs such as NFP with the most clear-cut evidence of effectiveness for families experiencing poverty.

References

Appel, H. (2008, January 7). Programs fight to cut infant death rate. *New York Daily News*. https://www.nydailynews.com/new-york/bronx/programs-fight-cut-infant-death-rate-article-1.341732

Avellar, S. A., & Supplee, L. H. (2013). Effectiveness of home visiting in improving child health and reducing child maltreatment. *Pediatrics*, *132*(Suppl. 2), S90–S99.

Barlow, A., Varipatis-Baker, E., Speakman, K., Ginsburg, G., Friberg, I., Goklish, N., Cowboy, B., Fields, P., Hastings, R., Pan, W., Reid, R., Santosham, M., & Walkup, J. (2006). Home-visiting intervention to improve child care among American Indian adolescent mothers: A randomized trial. *Archives of Pediatrics & Adolescent Medicine*, *160*(11), 1101–1107.

Burwick, A., Zaveri, H., Shang, L., Boller, K., Daro, D., & Strong, D. A. (2014). *Costs of early childhood home visiting: An analysis of programs implemented in the Supporting Evidence-Based Home Visiting to Prevent Child Maltreatment initiative*. Mathematica Policy Research. Retrieved May 8, 2021, from https://www.mathematica.org/~/media/publications/PDFs/earlychildhood/EBHV_costs.pdf

Cherniss, D. (1980). Treatment modalities. In S. Fraiberg (Ed.), *Clinical studies in infant mental health: The first year of life* (pp. 49–64). Basic Books.

Dodge, K. A., Goodman, W. B., Bai, Y., O'Donnell, K., & Murphy, R. A. (2019). Effect of a community agency–administered nurse home visitation program on program use and maternal and infant health outcomes: A randomized clinical trial. *JAMA Network Open*, *2*(11), Article e1914522. https://doi.org/10.1001/jamanetworkopen.2019.14522

Dodge, K. A., Goodman, W. B., Murphy, R. A., O'Donnell, K., Sato, J., & Guptill, S. (2014). Implementation and randomized controlled trial evaluation of universal postnatal nurse home visiting. *American Journal of Public Health*, *104*(Suppl. 1), S136–S143.

Filene, J. H., Kaminski, J. W., Valle, L. A., & Cachat, P. (2013). Components associated with home visiting program outcomes: A meta-analysis. *Pediatrics*, *132*(Suppl. 2), S100–S109.

Lewy, D. (2021). *Addressing racial and ethnic disparities in maternal and child health through home visiting programs.* Center for Health Care Strategies. Retrieved September 23, 2022, from https://www.chcs.org/media/Address ing-Racial-Ethnic-Disparities-Maternal-Child-Health-Home-Visiting-Programs.pdf

Lieberman, A. F. (2017). *The emotional life of the toddler.* Simon and Schuster.

Michalopoulos, C., Faucetta, K., Hill, C. J., Portilla, X. A., Burrell, L., Lee, H., Duggan, A., & Knox, V. (2019). *Impacts on family outcomes of evidence-based early childhood home visiting: Results from the mother and infant home visiting program evaluation. OPRE Report 2019-07.* Office of Planning, Research, and Evaluation, Administration for Children and Families, U.S. Department of Health and Human Services.

Miller, T. R. (2013). *Nurse-family partnership home visitation: Costs, outcomes, and return on investment.* Retrieved February 11, 2021, from https://iik.org/media/1259/costs_and_roi_report-pire.pdf

Miller, T. R. (2015). Projected outcomes of nurse-family partnership home visitation during 1996–2013, USA. *Prevention Science, 16*(6), 765–777.

New York State Department of Health. (2019). *How do I find the right program for my patient?* Retrieved February 11, 2021, from https://www.health.ny.gov/community/pregnancy/home_visiting_programs/provider.htm

Nurse–Family Partnership. (2021). *Annual report 2020.* Retrieved April 29, 2021, from https://www.nursefamilypartnership.org/about/annual-rep ort-2020/

Olds, D. L. (2006). The nurse–family partnership: An evidence-based preventive intervention. *Infant Mental Health Journal, 27*(1), 5–25.

Olds, D. L., Henderson Jr, C. R., Phelps, C., Kitzman, H., & Hanks, C. (1993). Effect of prenatal and infancy nurse home visitation on government spending. *Medical Care, 31*(2), 155–174.

Peacock, S., Konrad, S., Watson, E., Nickel, D., & Muhajarine, N. (2013). Effectiveness of home visiting programs on child outcomes: A systematic review. *BMC Public Health, 13*(1), 17.

Sweet, M. A., & Appelbaum, M. I. (2004). Is home visiting an effective strategy? A meta-analytic review of home visiting programs for families with young children. *Child Development, 75*(5), 1435–1456.

Weatherston, D. J., & Ribaudo, J. (2020). The Michigan infant mental health home visiting model. *Infant Mental Health Journal, 41*(2), 166–177.

Williams, D. R., Costa, M. V., Odunlami, A. O., & Mohammed, S. A. (2008). Moving upstream: How interventions that address the social determinants of health can improve health and reduce disparities. *Journal of Public Health Management and Practice, 14*(6), S8–S17. https://doi.org/10.1097/01.Phh.0000338382.36695.42

Wu, J., Dean, K. S., Rosen, Z., & Muennig, P. A. (2017). The cost-effectiveness analysis of nurse-family partnership in the United States. *Journal of Health Care for Poor and Underserved, 28*(4), 1578–1597.

4

Parent Training Programs

At most times of the year, but especially in this evening light of October, southwestern Vermont is an exceptionally beautiful place to be. Toward the east, the Green Mountains are aflame with slashes of vermilion, gold, and orange. Toward the west, the Taconics appear to be competing with the Green Mountains for the prize of most colorful mountain range. And in a valley in the middle, with views of both mountain ranges, nestles the town of Bennington.

The three occupants of a motel room close to downtown Bennington appear to be far more serious, paying little attention to the riot of color that is framed through the window. Edna and her son, Michael, live in the motel room and are being visited by Jenny, a family advocate at Sunrise Family Resource Center, one of Vermont's 15 parent–child centers. Parent–child centers in Vermont provide a set of core services—home visiting, early childhood services, parent education, playgroups, parent support groups, active support for families, community development, and information and referral to more specialized services. These centers, supported by the Vermont Department for Children and Families, offer these services at no charge to families.

"What led you to do that, Michael?" asks Jenny. "Could you tell me why you didn't log into your classes? What were you doing online at those times?"

Michael, his small frame seemingly swallowed by his jacket, shrugs but doesn't say anything, keeping his eyes on his blindingly white sneakers. Jenny turns to Edna and brings her into the conversation.

Investing in Children's Mental Health. Daniel Eisenberg and Ramesh Raghavan, Oxford University Press.
© Oxford University Press 2024. DOI: 10.1093/oso/9780190942014.003.0005

Michael is in middle school and has been absent, without his mother's knowledge, from online classes. The school has just sent Edna a letter threatening a truancy charge. Over the next half hour, Jenny and Edna discuss strategies to ensure reliable Internet connectivity within the motel room, set controls on Michael's laptop that will prevent him from accessing sites other than those directly relevant to his schoolwork, and establish a regular schedule for Michael's online learning. Some of the school's policies regarding expectations for attendance seem unclear to Edna, and Jenny helps Edna problem-solve ways to engage with the school so that she can better understand the policies.

Jenny is conducting a functional assessment—trying to determine what led to Michael's nonattendance so that she can better find ways to keep Michael engaged in school. In this assessment she is focusing not just on Michael, but on the relationship between Edna and Michael. By strengthening the bond between Edna and Michael, and by offering both of them various types of support, Jenny can help Edna better supervise Michael. The hope is that his behaviors will be reduced to the extent that he is no longer at risk of more serious delinquency.

The task, as is so often the case, is far more difficult than it sounds. Edna and Michael are unhoused, and the motel stay is a temporary shelter. Edna is worrying about finding a more permanent place to live, ensuring that her car is reliable enough for the upcoming winter so she can get to her job, and agonizing about what the pandemic will do to her job stability. Given all that is going on, the last thing she needs is a court date. Preoccupied by these survival concerns, she is frustrated by Michael's schooling troubles, and his seeming inability to appreciate the seriousness of his actions amid the precariousness of their lives—lives filled with the kinds of daily stress and uncertainty that seem at odds with the beauty of this region in Vermont, resplendent in its fall finery.

Disruptive Behavior Disorders and Parent Training Programs

Disruptive behavior disorders are a group of childhood conditions that have in common a loss of emotional or behavioral self-control on part of the child. Children with these conditions display defiance, may be irritable or surly, throw temper tantrums, and—in more severe instances—may engage in aggression toward other people, animals, or property. These disorders are complex; accurate identification needs to account for normal behaviors among children as they develop (indeed, the notion of "terrible twos" is commonplace within our society). Then there are other conditions that could explain some of the emotional outbursts such as a mood disorder. Accurate diagnosis also depends on the social context of such behaviors, and the cultural and gender-based norms that govern "acceptable" behavior in a particular society. These behaviors can have serious consequences for children, especially for youth of color who are at greater risk of entanglements with the juvenile justice system. Disruptive behaviors are a common reason for visits to child psychiatry units—an estimated 40%–60% of children presenting in these units are there for help with such behaviors (Steiner et al., 2017). This is why Jenny is visiting Edna and Michael. Michael's behaviors do not yet seem to rise to the level of a disruptive behavioral disorder, but truancy is a risk factor for the condition. By understanding and addressing the reasons behind Michael's absences from his classes, she is trying to forestall more serious problems that he might be at risk for as he grows up.

Until the 1960s, much of the treatment for disruptive behavior disorders was directed toward the child and used a psychodynamic treatment approach. However, beginning in the late 1960s, behavioral parent training emerged as a new paradigm that expanded the focus from the therapist–child dyad to also include the parent and began to equip parents with concrete tools that they could use to manage behaviors within the home (Graziano & Diament, 1992).

Any parent who has used time-out for a child who has thrown a temper tantrum, for example, is using a home-based, behavioral intervention. Parent training programs are simply extending and formalizing tools that many parents may have used during their child's toddlerhood. They are part of the same intervention paradigm and are based on the idea that the ways in which parents engage with their child, especially when it comes to disciplining their child, affect the manifestation and maintenance of the child's disruptive behaviors. Even though these programs are typically referred to as "parent" training, the term is not meant to be exclusionary. Any adult who has primary responsibility for the child can participate in such a program, even if they are not the child's birth parent.

Parent training programs are best thought of as a continuum of interventions spanning predominantly universal, prevention-focused models directed at all children to targeted interventions focused on addressing specific problematic child behaviors affecting some children. To some extent, all such programs teach parents ways to recognize problem behaviors, utilize interpersonal tools to manage such behaviors (e.g., ignoring the child, distraction, reinforcement, or punishment), and improve their parenting skills. These programs typically also teach parents to reinforce positive behaviors with attention and praise. Individual models of such programs conduct such training within places of work, schools, community or religious centers, or at home. Those programs that focus on children with serious behavior problems adopt a curative approach, while others that are more universal, and preventive, tend to emphasize caregiver capacity building in their approach.

There are several dozen well-established parent training programs, varying in their target age range and clinical needs of the child, the focus (parent, child, or system), the types of interventions used, and the manner of delivery. There are stand-alone parent training programs (such as The Incredible Years), and there are multicomponent interventions within which parenting skills are one component (such as in the home visiting programs that we discussed in Chapter 3, and multisystemic therapy that we will discuss in Chapter 6).

Some of these programs use exclusively behavioral strategies such as time-out, or reinforcing positive behaviors by praising them while ignoring tantrums, for example. This set of programs is termed by researchers as *behavioral* parent training approaches (Dumas, 1989; Serketich & Dumas, 1996). Many such programs are highly structured, are delivered by trained mental health or human services workers, utilize a written curriculum and training procedures (such as a program manual), and emphasize the teaching of specific parenting skills that can reduce parental frustration and avoid harsh punishment to the child. The target population for these types of programs are typically parents whose children have shown clear signs of a condition or a problem. Parents of children with developmental disorders, for example, benefit from behavioral parent training, as do parents whose child is at risk of entry into the juvenile justice system (Piquero et al., 2012).

Other programs, however, have less of a behavioral focus, emphasizing, for example, parent communication or education. Within these programs parents learn about good parenting practices, the limits and appropriateness of disciplining, better modes of interaction with their children, and early identification of problem behaviors (such as substance abuse) in their children. The work that Jenny is conducting with Edna and Michael falls more into this category. These programs are sometimes called *non-behavioral* parent training programs, which is a bit of a misnomer because they often include at least some behavioral strategies. In the Incredible Years program, for example, the Basic curriculum has a larger behavioral focus, while the Advance program, for parents who have successfully completed the Basic program, emphasizes problem-solving, communication, management of depression, family support, and the building of such capacities (Webster-Stratton & Reid, 2018). Both behavioral and non-behavioral programs are designed to change perceived problems in the child's behavior. The distinction lies in the magnitude and seriousness of the child's behavior, and in exactly what the programs do in order to change that behavior.

Some programs, while they focus on reducing problematic behaviors among children, also provide general parenting support to enhance parenting competencies, prevent the occurrence of problem behaviors among children, and, even more broadly, achieve the complete well-being of the child. For example, we spoke to staff members of a program in Elkhart County, Indiana, that deploys the Triple P program (Positive Parenting Program) for all parents in the county. Triple P of Elkhart County has an explicitly population-level focus and has worked within its community to move to an assets-based and systems-based approach to improving outcomes for children and families countywide. Their work has moved beyond parents who have been identified as being at risk for abuse or neglect. This approach is aligned to the Triple P intervention, which is based in a public health paradigm, with a tiered system of services according to the level of need across the spectrum in a community (Sanders, 1999). Triple P focuses on self-regulation as a unifying principle and involves teaching parents about desirable home environments, promoting child learning, appropriate discipline, ensuring reasonable expectations, and self-care, among other topics.

Finally, there are other programs that are less expert driven and more peer led. Parent support groups, for example, sometimes pair new parents, referred during their pregnancy, with more experienced parents to share information about various topics and resources. With all this complexity in exactly what the boundaries of "training" in parent training are, and how they are operationalized, whether policymakers should invest in them largely becomes a question regarding the availability of evidence around specific types of programs.

Evidence of Effectiveness

There have been at least three large quantitative reviews, or meta-analyses, that examine the effectiveness of parent training programs in changing disruptive child behaviors. The first meta-analysis examined 26 research studies on a non-behavioral parent training program called Parent Effectiveness Training (PET) (Cedar & Levant, 1990). PET is a type of parent training program that teaches specific communication skills to parents and thereby tries to change their knowledge, attitudes, behavior, and self-esteem, and, consequently, child behavior. This review found that PET produced effects in the "moderate" range on parents' attitudes and behavior. There were no immediate effects on children, which is not surprising because the focus of the treatment is on changing parents' competencies, and any resultant changes in parents' behaviors need time to translate into effects upon children. Too few of the studies had a long enough duration of follow up to determine if the program changed parents in some tangible way, and if these changes affected children's behavioral disruptions for the better.

Another review of a broader set of behavioral parent training programs found positive results for both child and parent outcomes (Serketich & Dumas, 1996). Effect sizes for children were large and indicated that children of participating parents were better off than 81% of children whose parents did not participate in a parent training program. Effects on parental adjustment (such as anxiety, stress, depression, and marital problems) were lower in magnitude but still significant, indicating that the benefits of participating in parent training accrue to both children and parents.

The third meta-analysis examined 63 research studies on behavioral and non-behavioral parent training programs (Lundahl et al., 2006). This review found that the effects of behavioral and non-behavioral parent training programs were roughly the same when it came to child behaviors, and that both of these types of parent training programs produced effects that were moderate in size immediately following treatment. When these groups were followed up for one year, the effects of behavioral parent training programs persisted but were weakened in the size of their effects—they were now in the small range. Too few non-behavioral programs followed up the groups for a year, so the persistence of effects of non-behavioral programs could not be studied by these authors.

In addition to the meta-analyses summarized above, a 2013 Cochrane Review examined 10 randomized control trials and three quasi-randomized trials of group-based parent training programs (Furlong et al., 2013). Overall, following parent training, child conduct problems were reduced, parents' mental health improved, and harsh or punitive parenting practices were reduced. Another review of four programs reported that behavioral and non-behavioral parent training programs seem to be equally effective in changing child behavior over the long run, though behavioral programs appear to produce their effects more rapidly (Högström et al., 2017).

Several specific parent training programs have demonstrated effectiveness in a variety of settings. The Blueprints registry lists one Model Plus parenting program, Generation Parent Management Training-Oregon (Forgatch & Gewirtz, 2017), and three other Model programs, including Nurse–Family Partnership, which we have discussed in Chapter 3 as an example of a home visiting program. Examples of other programs under the Promising category include Triple P (Sanders, 1999) and parent–child interaction therapy or PCIT (Hembree-Kigin & McNeil, 2013). Earlier in this chapter we mentioned a program called The Incredible Years, which is another Promising program according to Blueprints. This program has been extensively studied, and children—particularly younger children—participating in the program experience lower levels of problem behaviors, and higher levels of social competence. Their mothers also display reduced instances of negative parenting (Pidano & Allen, 2015). Early Risers is another program, not listed by Blueprints, that also appears to have demonstrated efficacy (August et al., 2001).

Economic Evidence

Reviews of parent training programs demonstrate cost-effectiveness. It costs approximately $2500 per family to reduce the average child's conduct problems from the clinical to the nonclinical range (Furlong et al., 2013). The authors described these program costs as modest, especially when compared with the long-term consequences—such as criminal justice involvement—of untreated childhood conduct problems. Britain's National Health Service (NHS) operates a Health Technology Assessment program that conducts cost-effectiveness studies of various programs used in the NHS. Their assessment of parent training found that each quality-adjusted life year (QALY) gained would cost between £38,393 and £6,288 ($48,017– $7,862, approximately) depending on the type of program delivery and setting, which is generally within the range that is considered cost-effective (Dretzke et al., 2005).

One study of the Incredible Years program found relatively high costs of administering the program within London schools—approximately £2,380 ($3,800) per child—but the program resulted in significant reductions in conduct problems, oppositional defiant disorder, and symptoms of ADHD, while showing increases of six months in reading age (Scott et al., 2010). Other studies have also shown cost-effectiveness for Incredible Years' parenting component; one study estimated a cost-effectiveness ratio of £73 ($42) for each one-point improvement on a scale of problem behaviors, for a total cost of £5,486 ($10,666) to bring a child with the highest score on the scale (indicating the worst outcome) to below the clinical cutoff point. Given the considerable costs that are imposed by problem behaviors to society if left unchecked, the authors concluded that this program represented good value for the money for public spending (Edwards et al., 2007). The estimates by the Washington State Institute for Public Policy (WSIPP) also make a case for investment in Incredible Years; total benefits from the program were $8,004 while net program costs amounted to $1,416, with a 59% chance that the benefits from the program will exceed costs.

Triple P has also been subject to economic evaluations at a population level, again with a positive result. Using a threshold analysis, authors of one study found that, in order to pay for itself, Triple P needs to prevent less than 1.5% of cases of conduct disorder (Mihalopoulos et al., 2007). This positive benefit relative to cost is maintained until the prevalence of conduct disorder falls below 7%, at which point it still is an effective intervention, but the costs are no longer lower than its cost savings. Another evaluation reported favorable costs per disability-adjusted life year averted among 5- to-9-year-olds followed through adulthood (Sampaio et al., 2018). Incremental cost-effectiveness ratios for Triple P in a group format were 1013 Australian dollars (approximately $720) per disability-adjusted life year averted, suggesting that Triple P represents a good investment at a population level. Estimates from WSIPP also support the wisdom of investments in the Triple P system—overall benefits ($2,375) were far greater than net program costs ($305), and there is a 71% chance that the program will produce more benefits than incur costs.

PCIT has also been subject to economic evaluations. A recent evaluation found an average cost of $1026 to treat one child (Goldfine et al., 2008). These investments produced impressive reductions in problem behaviors, resulting in a cost of between $22 and $101 to achieve a one-point reduction in various instruments quantifying the child's problem behaviors. WSIPP estimates suggest that the greatest benefits are seen for children involved in the child welfare system. For such children with histories of maltreatment, program costs of $1,727 produce benefits of $26,092 with a 96% chance that the program will produce greater benefits than costs. For these children, $1 invested in the program returns $15 in benefits.

Also, it seems clear that some key components of parent training are more effective than others. These components include those that increase positive parent–child interactions, teach communications skills, teach behavioral skills (such as time-out), emphasize consistency in parenting, and train parents by making them practice skills with their children during in-person training sessions (Wyatt Kaminski et al., 2008). It is far harder to conduct economic evaluations of components scattered across various programs and intervention styles than it is to conduct an evaluation of a packaged, manualized intervention. But it is likely that these effective elements, when delivered as part of "usual care," may prove to be a cost-effective way to build parenting capacity. We return to this theme of core components repeatedly in this book.

Equity Considerations

Parenting is a distinctly culturally bounded experience. Unless you happen to be a mental health professional well versed in the parenting literature, the way in which you parent is perhaps largely modeled around the ways in which you were parented yourself. And the childhoods we know best are our own, so it is natural to assume that everyone else's experience is similar. For this reason, parenting interventions need to be especially attuned to issues of culture, both in terms of macro-culture (such as incorporating norms of *familismo* and *respeto* within Latinx families [Calzada, 2010]), but also micro-culture, honoring uniquely intrafamilial ways of raising children. This is especially the case if the development of these programs occurred within a predominantly European-American culture. The best programs thread this needle skillfully, because the consequences of ignoring the highly personal nature of parenting can lead to program ineffectiveness.

This is perhaps why some prior studies and reviews have identified the concerning fact that the effects of parent training programs are weaker among families who have low incomes or belong to ethnic minority cultures (Griner & Smith, 2006; Lundahl et al., 2006). Social disadvantage is sometimes accompanied by a lack of social support, the need to stop treatment early because of other pressing needs, and the lack of customizable treatment that is uniquely relevant to the needs of families living in poverty. For such families, individually delivered parent training appears to be more effective than group-delivered parent training (Lundahl et al., 2006).

Tailoring parenting programs for participants belonging to different cultures is especially important. Scholars have suggested that programs need to be linguistically competent, include shared cultural beliefs about parenting, and incorporate cultural explanations for behavioral phenomena rather than seek to refute them (Griner & Smith, 2006). In these ways, the cultural adaptation or tailoring of parenting interventions can improve their acceptance and, consequently, their effectiveness. Such adaptations might increase the costs of the program but are important to consider in the interests of delivering effective programs to families that need them the most. The programs named in this chapter—including Parent Management Training Oregon, Incredible Years, and Triple P—have each been culturally adapted in various ways to better meet the needs of diverse populations. These types of adaptations generally lead to greater effectiveness (van Mourik et al., 2017).

Conclusions

There are a variety of parenting programs with robust evidence of effectiveness and cost-effectiveness, including both programs for children with clinical needs and for more general populations. Many of these programs have achieved these outcomes in diverse populations, as a result of careful adaptations and built-in flexibility in their approach. Nevertheless, some reviews suggest that parent training programs have generally shown weaker effects for families experiencing poverty, indicating a continued need for these programs to account for the context in which children and families are living.

References

August, G. J., Realmuto, G. M., Hektner, J. M., & Bloomquist, M. L. (2001). An integrated components preventive intervention for aggressive elementary school children: The Early Risers program. *Journal of Consulting and Clinical Psychology, 69*(4), 614–626.

Calzada, E. J. (2010). Bringing culture into parent training with Latinos. *Cognitive and Behavioral Practice, 17*(2), 167–175.

Cedar, B., & Levant, R. F. (1990). A meta-analysis of the effects of parent effectiveness training. *The American Journal of Family Therapy, 18*(4), 373–384.

Dretzke, J., Frew, E., Davenport, C., Barlow, J., Stewart-Brown, S., Sandercock, J., Bayliss, S., Raftery, J., Hyde, C., & Taylor, R. (2005). The effectiveness and cost-effectiveness of parent training/education programmes for the treatment of conduct disorder, including oppositional defiant disorder, in children. *Health Technology Assessment, 9*(50), iii, ix–x, 1–233.

Dumas, J. E. (1989). Treating antisocial behavior in children: Child and family approaches. *Clinical Psychology Review, 9*(2), 197–222.

Edwards, R. T., Céilleachair, A., Bywater, T., Hughes, D. A., & Hutchings, J. (2007). Parenting programme for parents of children at risk of developing conduct disorder: Cost effectiveness analysis. *British Medical Journal, 334*(7595), 682.

Forgatch, M. S., & Gewirtz, A. H. (2017). The evolution of the Oregon model of parent management training. In J. R. Weisz & A. E. Kazdin (Eds.), *Evidence-based psychotherapies for children and adolescents, third edition* (pp. 85–102). The Guilford Press.

Furlong, M., McGilloway, S., Bywater, T., Hutchings, J., Smith, S. M., & Donnelly, M. (2013). Cochrane review: Behavioural and cognitive-behavioural group-based parenting programmes for early-onset conduct problems in children aged 3 to 12 years (Review). *Evidence Based Child Health, 8*(2), 318–692.

Goldfine, M. E., Wagner, S. M., Branstetter, S. A., & McNeil, C. B. (2008). Parent-child interaction therapy: An examination of cost-effectiveness. *Journal of Early and Intensive Behavior Intervention, 5*(1), 119–141.

Graziano, A. M., & Diament, D. M. (1992). Parent behavioral training: An examination of the paradigm. *Behavior Modification, 16*(1), 3–38.

Griner, D., & Smith, T. B. (2006). Culturally adapted mental health intervention: A meta-analytic review. *Psychotherapy: Theory, Research, Practice, Training, 43*(4), 531–548.

Hembree-Kigin, T. L., & McNeil, C. B. (2013). *Parent–child interaction therapy.* Springer Science & Business Media.

Högström, J., Olofsson, V., Özdemir, M., Enebrink, P., & Stattin, H. (2017). Two-year findings from a national effectiveness trial: Effectiveness of behavioral and non-behavioral parenting programs. *Journal of Abnormal Child Psychology, 45*(3), 527–542.

Lundahl, B., Risser, H. J., & Lovejoy, M. C. (2006). A meta-analysis of parent training: Moderators and follow-up effects. *Clinical Psychology Review, 26*(1), 86–104.

Mihalopoulos, C., Sanders, M. R., Turner, K. M., Murphy-Brennan, M., & Carter, R. (2007). Does the Triple P–positive parenting program provide value for money? *Australian & New Zealand Journal of Psychiatry, 41*(3), 239–246.

Pidano, A. E., & Allen, A. R. (2015). The Incredible Years series: A review of the independent research base. *Journal of Child and Family Studies, 24*(7), 1898–1916.

Piquero, A. R., & Jennings, W. G. (2012). Parent training and the prevention of crime. In D. P. Farrington & B. C. Welsh (Eds.), *The Oxford Handbook of Crime Prevention* (pp. 89–101). Oxford University Press.

Sampaio, F., Barendregt, J. J., Feldman, I., Lee, Y. Y., Sawyer, M. G., Dadds, M. R., Scott, J. G., & Mihalopoulos, C. (2018). Population cost-effectiveness of the Triple P parenting programme for the treatment of conduct disorder: An economic modelling study. *European Child & Adolescent Psychiatry, 27*(7), 933–944.

Sanders, M. R. (1999). Triple P-Positive Parenting Program: Towards an empirically validated multilevel parenting and family support strategy for the prevention of behavior and emotional problems in children. *Clinical Child and Family Psychology Review, 2*(2), 71–90.

Scott, S., Sylva, K., Doolan, M., Price, J., Jacobs, B., Crook, C., & Landau, S. (2010). Randomised controlled trial of parent groups for child antisocial behaviour targeting multiple risk factors: The SPOKES project. *Journal of Child Psychology and Psychiatry, 51*(1), 48–57.

Serketich, W. J., & Dumas, J. E. (1996). The effectiveness of behavioral parent training to modify antisocial behavior in children: A meta-analysis. *Behavior Therapy, 27*(2), 171–186.

Steiner, H., Daniels, W., Stadler, C., & Kelly, M. (2017). *Disruptive behavior: Development, psychopathology, crime, & treatment.* Oxford University Press.

van Mourik, K., Crone, M. R., de Wolff, M. S., & Reis, R. (2017). Parent training programs for ethnic minorities: A meta-analysis of adaptations and effect. *Prevention Science, 18*(1), 95–105.

Webster-Stratton, C., & Reid, M. J. (2017). The Incredible Years parents, teachers, and children training series: A multifaceted treatment approach for young children with conduct problems. In J. R. Weisz & A. E. Kazdin (Eds.), *Evidence-based psychotherapies for children and adolescents* (3rd ed., pp. 122–141). The Guilford Press.

Wyatt Kaminski, J., Valle, L. A., Filene, J. H., & Boyle, C. L. (2008). A meta-analytic review of components associated with parent training program effectiveness. *Journal of Abnormal Child Psychology, 36*(4), 567–589.

5

School-Based Social-Emotional Learning (SEL) Programs

In recent years, educators in the United States and other countries have paid increasing attention to children's social-emotional learning (SEL), as a complement to traditional academic skills. SEL consists of five types of skills related to emotions, behaviors, and interpersonal relationships, according to the Collaborative for Academic, Social, and Emotional Learning (CASEL) (Weissberg et al., 2015); these are self-awareness, self-regulation, interpersonal awareness, relationship skills, and positive decision-making.

SEL has strong links to mental health. It emphasizes steps for dealing with emotions, much like many approaches to mental health therapy: recognizing, understanding, labeling, expressing, and regulating emotions (Brackett et al., 2015). SEL skills during childhood predict the later onset of mental health conditions such as depression, as well as a wide range of academic, social, behavioral, and other health outcomes in later childhood, adolescence, and adulthood (Jones, Greenberg, et al., 2015).

SEL in the Cleveland Metropolitan School District

The home of SEL in the Cleveland Metropolitan School District's is located on the 18th floor of a building in the heart of downtown Cleveland. From their offices the sweeping panorama of the city and Lake Erie match the enduring vision through which their

Investing in Children's Mental Health. Daniel Eisenberg and Ramesh Raghavan, Oxford University Press.
© Oxford University Press 2024. DOI: 10.1093/oso/9780190942014.003.0006

leadership team—starting with the district's chief executive officer, Eric Gordon—has steadily ingrained SEL into its culture. While the entire state of Ohio has recently adopted SEL standards for its schools, the Cleveland district is unique in its long-standing, deliberate approach to SEL.

In 2008 Gordon created an organization, Humanware, as part of the district's response to a school shooting that occurred the previous year. Bill Stencil, who had been working in the district on programs related to mental health crises, was installed as the director of Humanware and has provided steady leadership for these activities since that time. The efforts began with a strengthening of physical protections in the schools—"hardware," as they like to call it—and Gordon, Stencil, and their colleagues argued successfully for a parallel increase in efforts to address social and emotional skills and challenges, hence the name Humanware. The development of Humanware followed years of groundwork by Stencil and others implementing district programs such as Rapid Response for mental health–related crises, which began in the early 1990s. With the creation of Humanware, the district invested heavily in the PATHS® curriculum (Promoting Alternative Thinking Strategies) as a universal SEL program for elementary schools. This early investment was boosted by the availability of federal stimulus funds through the American Reinvestment and Recovery Act.

A look inside the Cleveland schools offers a sense of the successes and remaining challenges. Accompanied by Stencil and his colleague Lathardus Goggins, we first visit Memorial Elementary, which has a 100% black student population. On a cool, cloudy day in spring 2019, the old, handsome brick school building with sparse grounds looks at home in its working-class neighborhood. Upon entering the building, we are greeted warmly by office staff members and respectfully by older students who are stationed in the hallways to alert passersby about testing in nearby classrooms.

We first observe a first grade classroom taught by Jillian Ahrens. She is one of the most active promoters and users of PATHS in the district and is a vice president of the Cleveland Teachers Union. The classroom walls display PATHS posters right under the American flag and pledge of allegiance. One poster shows the three steps for calming down, a staple of the program. In today's lesson, the students look at various facial expressions and situations related to emotions: surprise, and comfortable versus uncomfortable. Examples include a boy tripping over a dog, a girl finding a dollar bill on the ground, and a boy unwrapping a gift box with a football inside. They talk about the word "expect" and how it relates to surprises and feelings. They review the turtle technique for calming down when an uncomfortable surprise occurs—this technique involves recognizing emotions and going into one's "shell" to calm down and think calming thoughts before confronting a situation. The teacher, Ms. Ahrens, has a turtle puppet on her hand during this discussion. The lesson illustrates the connection with academic content for much of the PATHS curriculum—in this case, vocabulary and storytelling as part of the language arts curriculum. PATHS gives words for children to recognize and describe their thoughts and feelings with, and it promotes a problem-solving mindset. At the end of the lesson, the students personalize the words and ideas by drawing their own faces experiencing comfortable and uncomfortable surprises.

After the lesson, Ms. Ahrens debriefs us with the principal, Maria Dinkins. They share stories about students whose behavior and confidence benefited from PATHS. For example, a fourth grader was once dropped off at school on a day when school was out, and nobody was there to help her. She used her calming and problem-solving skills and walked to a nearby Burger King and asked them to call her parents. Principal Dinkins ensures that all teachers train and retrain in PATHS on a regular basis, and they participate in many other training opportunities related to SEL. She credits PATHS and other SEL efforts in the school's recent declines in student suspensions; their rates are now among the lowest of the 18 schools in their network of peer schools in the district.

We then visit Clark Elementary, a school with predominantly Latinx and black students in a low-income, industrial neighborhood on the west side of Cleveland. We observe the second-grade classroom of Darmaris Sanchez, who has received district-wide recognition for her teaching. The PATHS lesson starts with the students sitting on a rug, except for one boy in a chair, the PATHS "kid of the day." The other students are invited to give him compliments, and they say things such as "he plays nicely" and "he always asks if he wants to play something." When asked to compliment himself, the boy softly says that he always keeps his room clean at home. The class then discusses a word of the day, "malicious." They talk about how feeling malicious is normal; all feelings are okay to experience. What is not okay is acting out of anger and maliciousness, Ms. Sanchez emphasizes. They also talk about uncomfortable versus comfortable feelings. Malicious is an uncomfortable feeling—a warning sign. The opposite of malicious is kind. Being kind makes you feel good. Kindness should be shared with everyone, not just friends and family. Ms. Sanchez points out how she treats everyone kindly around the school, no matter who they are. She asks the children to imagine a world full of random acts of kindness versus a world full of maliciousness. Which world would they want to live in?

In debriefings with the assistant principal, Cedric McEachron, and the principal, Amanda Rodriguez, they both note that relationship building is a priority at their school, and SEL has been central to those efforts. Just a few minutes earlier, McEachron notes, a child had a temper tantrum in his office but was able to calm down; this child probably would not have been able to do that in the past, he notes. The school sets high expectations and recognizes teachers for doing well with PATHS. When they hire teachers, they ask about their openness to different approaches and their perspective on discipline and social and emotional development. Their school has many SEL-related pieces in addition to PATHS, and they view SEL for their teachers and other staff members as important too. They have a teacher well-being program, CARE (Cultivating Awareness and Resilience in Education), which is provided by Creating Resilience for Educators, Administrators, and Teachers (CREATE) (https://createforeducation.org/care/); CARE is an evidence-based program that includes a two-day workshop plus follow-up sessions and weekly emails (Jennings et al., 2017). Clark Elementary has also implemented the Community Approach to Learning Mindfully (CALM) program (Harris et al., 2016), which holds brief yoga sessions for teachers and other staff members before the school day starts.

Principal Rodriguez became an advocate for PATHS and SEL based on a personal experience. Her son was five years old at the time that PATHS was introduced in Cleveland. He threw a tantrum in the back of the car when they passed a McDonald's and she did not agree to his request to stop there. After a couple minutes the tantrum unexpectedly stopped, and she looked back to see him "turtling"—using the turtle technique to calm down. The incident moved her so much that she started pushing the next day for the greater use of PATHS and SEL in her school.

Both the principal and assistant principal acknowledge that challenges remain for their school's efforts to promote social and emotional support and development. They speak of the difficulty in engaging parents and families in the effort. They often have low turnout when they hold events or workshops for families, many of whom are struggling to handle a variety of life challenges. Principal Rodriguez also points to the continual struggle of adding enough resources to keep up with the increasing mental health needs of students, who are more likely to have experienced trauma than previous cohorts.

Based on our observations and interviews, the relatively successful implementation of PATHS and other SEL initiatives in Cleveland appears to be driven by a few key factors. First, the district has had champions of SEL at all levels: at the district level, with Gordon as the visionary leader and Stencil and his Humanware team as the tireless organizers and implementers, and at the school level, with exemplary principals and teachers such as those at Memorial and Clark. And these champions beget champions, through their hiring decisions and the encouragement and recognition they provide to teachers and other staff members. Second, the district underwent a careful process of planning and gaining widespread buy-in when they created Humanware. In 2007–2008 they did a yearlong process to vet and select SEL programs. They used a 13-question matrix to assess the strengths and weaknesses of several alternatives, with assistance from CASEL. The planning and selection process was inclusive of not only district leadership but also the teacher's union. They chose PATHS for several reasons: decades of evidence; roots in child development and psychological theory; coverage of pre-K through fifth, with scaffolding of skills over that range; and the emphasis on teaching skills carefully before asking people to apply them (Kusché & Greenberg, 2012). They chose to train all their teachers, rather than just a specialized subset of staff members, so that SEL would be embedded in their culture and would reach students throughout the day.

Another key ingredient for success has been a consistent monitoring of outcomes and evolution of best practices. The district remains in regular contact with the PATHS program developer, Mark Greenberg, and the leader of the training organization (SEL Worldwide), Dorothy Morelli. They conduct continuous monitoring of outcomes, in partnership with the American Institutes for Research (AIR), using the Conditions for Learning (CFL) assessment twice a year for all students. The schools with the best CFL scores also tend to have the best academic test scores, according to Stencil. They also track other indicators of success such as attendance, referrals to the principal, and suspensions. In addition, they maintain a continuous push for training new teachers and other staff members and retraining experienced teachers and staff. With support from SEL Worldwide the training is done by people within the district, which means they are not relying on outside trainers. Lastly, they have embraced many other SEL-related initiatives, aside from their core programs (PATHS and another well-known program, Second Step), infusing the values in the schools' cultures. Examples include SEL programs for adult staff members and a new focus on restorative justice.

Everyone we interviewed in Cleveland acknowledges there are still challenges and room for improvement. While schools such as Memorial and Clark are thriving in their implementation of PATHS and SEL more broadly, as of 2019 there were only about 15 such schools district-wide that are recognized as "model" PATHS schools. Stencil and Goggins believe that at many other schools the principals or teachers have not fully embraced SEL because it is not central to how they were trained as educators. There are no easy answers for how to get these other schools to implement and sustain PATHS and SEL more broadly. The launch of the Say Yes program in Cleveland in 2019 offers a new source of optimism, however, as it is helping to bring another wave of resources and attention to SEL. Cleveland was selected as one of a small number of communities nationwide in the initial cohort for this ambitious initiative to increase graduation rates and improve the learning environment in schools.

Broader Trends and Lessons

Cleveland is but one example of a larger movement toward SEL over approximately the past 30 years in the United States. Experts we interviewed point to several factors to explain the rising enthusiasm for SEL. First, SEL is consistent with basic principles of education that have been widely appreciated for many decades, only under different names. As one expert noted, SEL is simply an essential feature of good teaching: high-quality interactions and relationships with kids that undergird conversations about academic content. Second, a critical mass of research evidence has been built, including hundreds of evaluation studies with generally favorable findings. Third, there is a growing appreciation in society more broadly for the importance of "soft skills" in determining success in school and careers. Several prominent scholars and their colleagues have brought these ideas into popular and policy conversations, such as Angela Duckworth's emphasis on *grit* (Duckworth et al., 2007), Carol Dweck's study of *growth mindsets* (Dweck, 2017), and James Heckman's focus on *non-cognitive* skills (Heckman & Kautz, 2012). The journalist Paul Tough has expanded this audience further with his bestselling book, *How Children Succeed*, which synthesizes this collection of research and weaves it with stories of young people and their families, schools, and other organizations supporting youth development. The Aspen Institute National Commission on Social, Emotional, and Academic Development compiled an uplifting summary and call to action based on this growing appreciation for social and emotional skills in the United States (Aspen Institute, 2018).

The economist David Deming offers a compelling theory for exactly *how* social and emotional skills enhance career success (Deming, 2017). He hypothesizes and finds empirical support for a specific mechanism by which interpersonal and emotional skills determine the ability to work effectively in teams, which involves "trading" work activities based on one's relative advantages in skills. In a dynamic, flexible professional environment, this requires effective interpersonal communication and understanding among team members.

Evidence of Effectiveness and Cost-Effectiveness

There is a growing base of evidence indicating a range of positive effects for SEL programs. A widely cited meta-analysis from 2011 reviewed over 200 school-based SEL programs and found significant improvements in social and emotional skills, attitudes, behaviors, and academic performance (Durlak et al., 2011). A more recent meta-analysis built on the earlier one by focusing on the duration of effects (Taylor et al., 2017); they reviewed 82 studies, mostly randomized control trials (RCTs), of school-based SEL programs with outcomes six months or more after the intervention period and again found significant effects, mostly in the small-to-medium range, for nearly all of the outcomes they examined. These positive effects were present across socioeconomic status and race/ethnicity; there were no significant differences in effect sizes across school populations that were predominantly students of color, predominantly white students, or a more even mix, or across school populations that were predominantly lower income, predominantly higher income, or a more even mix.

Although the meta-analyses are frequently cited to support the effectiveness of SEL on a broad level, all programs do not have equal levels of evidence. Two programs, PATHS and Positive Action, are recognized as Model programs in the Blueprints registry, each with multiple high-quality randomized trials demonstrating effectiveness. Along with these two programs, several other programs are highlighted in the *Handbook of Social and Emotional Learning* as meeting criteria for "what works": at the preschool level, Incredible Years; at the elementary level, Second Step, Caring School Community, and Responsive Classroom; and at the middle school level, Life Skills Training and Responding in Peaceful and Positive Ways (RIPP). At the high school level, no program meets the full criteria for "what works," but several are designated as promising. At the postsecondary level, mindfulness interventions are recognized as a category of program with consistently positive results. Many other programs are in the "promising" category at all levels of education.

Although there is now plenty of evidence supporting the effectiveness of SEL programs, there are still important limitations in the research. Outcomes are often reported by teachers or focused on subjective skills rather than objective behaviors. As in the general child development literature, fade-out of initial effects is a major concern. The meta-analysis noted above by Taylor and colleagues addresses this issue to some degree, but they found that most studies had no more than one- or two-year follow-up periods. In addition, the mechanisms for positive effects of SEL programs are not clear in many cases. Relatedly, most programs are integrated with academic content, making it difficult to quantify the degree to which SEL-specific skills are responsible for academic improvements.

Based on the generally encouraging evidence for the effectiveness of SEL programs, some analysts have extrapolated to an economic case. The Washington State Institute for Public Policy (WSIPP) estimates that both Positive Action and PATHS have very favorable benefit–cost differentials per participant: $14,002 benefits versus $444 costs for Positive Action, and $7,487 versus $360 for PATHS. Another report uses the best available data to assess the benefit–cost ratios for several prominent SEL programs (Belfield et al., 2015): 4Rs, Positive Action, Life Skills Training, Second Step, Responsive Classroom, and Social and Emotional Training. They find favorable benefit–cost ratios for this set of programs as a whole, and they note that any variation in their results across programs should not be overemphasized, as it can result from differing availability of measures that are translatable into economic benefits. For Positive Action, for example, they estimate benefits of $2,580 per participant compared with costs of $510 per participant. As they discuss in their report, these numbers are based on a number of uncertain assumptions, and there are important opportunities to improve data and research in this area. Similarly, Jones and colleagues (2015) discuss the strengths and limitations of economic evidence for SEL programs and identify the biggest challenge and area for improvement: determining the longer run economic value of short-term outcomes commonly produced by SEL programs. This is particularly difficult for younger children, because the short-term outcomes are so far removed in time from economic consequences such as employment and earnings in adulthood.

Implementation Challenges (Have We Reached a Plateau?)

Despite the rising enthusiasm for SEL programs, the experts we interviewed agreed that changes in practice and policy have been modest relative to the full potential of SEL. This view is consistent with the available data on the national penetration of SEL programs. Probably the most widely used SEL-related program is Positive Behavior Interventions and Supports (PBIS), which is present in an estimated 25,000 schools in the United States. PBIS is a general framework to address behavior and school climate, but the use of this framework does not necessarily imply a thorough implementation, nor any kind of comprehensive SEL curriculum. Furthermore, 25,000 is still less than a quarter of the more than 100,000 elementary and secondary schools in the United States. For more structured and specific SEL programs with the strongest evidence of effectiveness—such as PATHS and Positive Action—the national penetration is much lower, at less than 3% in each case, based on numbers available on the programs' websites.

The relatively low penetration of SEL programs is not entirely surprising when one considers the barriers to implementation. Perhaps the biggest barrier is simply that educators, in an era of school accountability and standardized testing, are reluctant to dedicate the curriculum time necessary to implement comprehensive programs such as PATHS and Positive Action. Even when these types of programs are used, they are less impactful when they are not fully implemented. Another implementation challenge is that some of the most effective programs, such as PATHS, insist on intensive in-person training for teachers and school professionals who deliver the program. This attention to high-quality implementation maximizes the chances of positive outcomes but requires considerable investments of time from both trainers and trainees. Again, the reluctance of schools to devote substantial time and resources becomes a barrier.

"Kernels": A New Alternative

Stephanie Jones and colleagues propose a "kernel" approach as a solution to the limited space in school curricula (Jones & Bouffard, 2012). They have looked for common elements, or "common denominators," in SEL programs with positive outcomes. They hypothesize that these common elements are likely to be the active ingredients and examine how to implement them in as light and flexible ways as possible. They note that this approach is well received by practitioners in schools, who appreciate the agency and flexibility. This approach yields a variety of ways to integrate into the full school context, rather than just classrooms and formal curricula.

The kernel approach has been piloted with promising results at a small number of sites throughout the country. In the Twin Rivers Unified District in Sacramento, Christopher Williams from the Ecological Approaches to Social Emotional Learning (EASEL) Laboratory oversaw a two-year project to implement the approach at some of the schools. In the first year they conducted a series of training sessions for the teachers—around 70 in total, from two elementary schools plus special education teachers throughout the district. In the second year they conducted a randomized trial to evaluate the impacts. At each training they introduced 10–12 kernels and solicited feedback from the teachers.

Mr. Williams has been working in education and mental health for about 20 years and sees the kernel approach as a major advance. He says this is the first time he has seen that every single professional is using skills and activities from a training, and most of them are using something every school day. He believes the kernels approach is "light years ahead of the boxed curricula." In his view, the more structured curricula sometimes convey implicitly that soft skills are separate and less important than academic skills, whereas the kernels are more empowering to the teachers and are practical and easy to implement. The 5–10 minutes required for many kernels are worthwhile investments of time by teachers because they allow students to regain focus. He notes that one sixth grade teacher in Sacramento reports that her students are now requesting community circles (one of the kernels) after recess to resolve or process conflicts, and a first-grade teacher says that her kids will not leave for the day until they have had a chance to play zip-zap-zop, a fast-paced game that promotes a sense of fun and cooperation within a group. The participating schools have seen approximately 75% fewer referrals to the principal and 30%–40% fewer suspensions in the previous year, and Mr. Williams attributes much of those changes to the implementation of kernels.

Another site using kernels is the summer program, Horizons at Green Farms Academy in Bridgeport, Connecticut. The Horizons program helps students from low-income families and students who are struggling academically. It takes place over six weeks during the summer, plus 11 Saturdays interspersed across the school year. The students all come from the Bridgeport district, which is one of the lowest performing in the state. Their students are roughly 60% Latino, 40% black. SEL is core to their program, which reflects the vision of Joe Aleardi, their director. In collaboration with the EASEL Lab, they have implemented kernels with a focus on a new SEL area each year. Examples of SEL areas by grade level include: stop-and-think power in kindergarten, focus power in first grade, remember power in second grade, and relationship skills in fifth grade. They are continuing to build additional skills for middle school and high school students. They had good results from pre-post evaluations after the first two summers in 2017 and 2018, according to Aleardi. Kernels work well for their context, where they have just six uninterrupted weeks with the kids each year. Teachers have flexibility in how they deliver SEL skills. They are encouraged to emphasize their grade level's focus area, but they can also draw from a much broader "playbook" provided by the EASEL Lab or discover SEL activities on their own. The kernels approach is clearly attracting followers in the education world, and it will be interesting to see whether it starts to replace more traditional, structured programs on a wider scale. In a sense, the use of kernels is not a completely new approach in SEL, as it has been present in many respects in some of the larger programs. For example, PATHS includes a variety of kernels such as posters in the hallways, Problem-Solving sheets in the principal and counselor's office, and the turtle technique. At a minimum, it seems likely that the kernels approach is encouraging more flexibility in thinking about the increments in which SEL skills and practices are implemented in schools.

Equity Considerations

In general, a variety of evidence indicates that SEL programs can be effective across a range of student populations with varying racial/ethnic and socioeconomic compositions. Of course, this general statement does not guarantee that each specific SEL program will be effective in each specific community. The evidence specific for each program must be considered in its own right, and adaptations to local culture and context may be needed in some cases. It is encouraging that some of the most notable success stories that we have identified—such as Cleveland, Bridgeport, and Sacramento—have benefited school populations with high proportions of students of color and lower income families. All indications are that SEL has an important role to play in promoting greater equity in education and well-being for children. Additional research and policy efforts will be needed to tap this full potential.

Summary

In light of the enthusiasm, successes, and innovations described in this chapter, SEL programs clearly represent a promising investment with exciting opportunities for growth. There is a solid base of evidence that some programs have short-term benefits, at a minimum. Those short-term benefits alone may be sufficient to justify the modest costs associated with implementing programs. For this investment to reach a wider scale in the United States and beyond, however, it is important to understand more fully the longer-term benefits, the mechanisms of action, and the most efficient training and implementation strategies. The recent attention to school safety may help sustain interest in this area, as policymakers and other stakeholders increasingly recognize the important role that schools play in young people's social and emotional development.

References

Aspen Institute. (2018). *From a nation at risk to a nation at hope: Recommendations from the National Commission on Social, Emotional, and Academic Development.* http://nationathope.org/wp-content/uploads/2018_aspen_final-report_full_webversion.pdf

Belfield, C., Bowden, A. B., Klapp, A., Levin, H., Shand, R., & Zander, S. (2015). The economic value of social and emotional learning. *Journal of Benefit-Cost Analysis, 6*(3), 508–544.

Brackett, M. A., Elbertson, N. A., & Rivers, S. E. (2015). Applying theory to the development of approaches to SEL. In J. A. Durlak, C. E. Domitrovich, R. P. Weissberg, & T. P. Gullotta (Eds.), *Handbook of social and emotional learning: Research and practice* (pp. 20–32). The Guilford Press.

Deming, D. J. (2017). The growing importance of social skills in the labor market. *The Quarterly Journal of Economics, 132*(4), 1593–1640.

Duckworth, A. L., Peterson, C., Matthews, M. D., & Kelly, D. R. (2007). Grit: Perseverance and passion for long-term goals. *Journal of Personality and Social Psychology, 92*(6), 1087–1101.

Durlak, J. A., Weissberg, R. P., Dymnicki, A. B., Taylor, R. D., & Schellinger, K. B. (2011). The impact of enhancing students' social and emotional learning: A meta-analysis of school-based universal interventions. *Child Development, 82*(1), 405–432.

Dweck, C. S. (2017). The journey to children's mindsets—And beyond. *Child Development Perspectives, 11*(2), 139–144.

Harris, A. R., Jennings, P. A., Katz, D. A., Abenavoli, R. M., & Greenberg, M. T. (2016). Promoting stress management and wellbeing in educators: Feasibility and efficacy of a school-based yoga and mindfulness intervention. *Mindfulness, 7*(1), 143–154.

Heckman, J. J., & Kautz, T. (2012). Hard evidence on soft skills. *Labour Economics, 19*(4), 451–464.

Jennings, P. A., Brown, J. L., Frank, J. L., Doyle, S., Oh, Y., Davis, R., Rasheed, D., DeWeese, A., DeMauro, A. A., & Cham, H. (2017). Impacts of the CARE for Teachers program on teachers' social and emotional competence and classroom interactions. *Journal of Educational Psychology, 109*(7), 1010–1028.

Jones, D. E., Greenberg, M., & Crowley, M. (2015). Early social-emotional functioning and public health: The relationship between kindergarten social competence and future wellness. *American Journal of Public Health, 105*(11), 2283–2290.

Jones, D. E., Karoly, L. A., Crowley, D. M., & Greenberg, M. T. (2015). Considering valuation of noncognitive skills in benefit-cost analysis of programs for children. *Journal of Benefit-Cost Analysis, 6*(3), 471–507.

Jones, S. M., & Bouffard, S. M. (2012). Social and emotional learning in schools: From programs to strategies and commentaries. *Social Policy Report, 26*(4), 1–33.

Kusché, C., & Greenberg, M. (2012). The PATHS curriculum: Promoting emotional literacy, prosocial behavior, and caring classrooms. In S. Jimerson, A. Nickerson, M. J. Mayer, & M. J. Furlong (Eds.), *Handbook of School Violence and Safety* (pp. 435–446). Routledge.

Taylor, R. D., Oberle, E., Durlak, J. A., & Weissberg, R. P. (2017). Promoting positive youth development through school-based social and emotional learning interventions: A meta-analysis of follow-up effects. *Child Development, 88*(4), 1156–1171.

Weissberg, R. P., Durlak, J. A., Domitrovich, C. E., & Gullotta, T. P. (2015). Social and emotional learning: Past, present, and future. In J. A. Durlak, C. E. Domitrovich, R. P. Weissberg, & T. P. Gullotta (Eds.), *Handbook of social and emotional learning: Research and practice* (pp. 3–19). The Guilford Press.

6

Multisystemic Therapy

The Fluorescent Light Bulb Not Everyone Is Using

Multisystemic therapy (MST) represents an ideal case, in many respects, for understanding the best investments in children's mental health. It has a long history of research, evaluation, and dissemination throughout the United States and other countries, and it is a radical departure from traditional approaches to mental and behavioral health among troubled children and youth. Despite its relative success in spreading as an evidence-based practice, it still only reaches a small fraction of the population who would likely benefit. Keller Strother, the director and cofounder of MST Services, the organization that promotes and facilitates the dissemination of the program, makes the analogy with the fluorescent light bulb. Much as fluorescent bulbs have taken decades to become the standard, MST is an innovation that is clearly better than preexisting alternatives but has been adopted slowly, in large part because it is so different from prevailing standards and interests.

MST is an intensive set of treatment services designed to help youth and their families with severe mental and behavioral health needs, for whom usual solutions are not working. MST is delivered in home, school, and other community settings by a team of therapists and focuses on youth who have engaged in violent or illegal behaviors and are at risk of removal from their homes and being sent to foster care or residential care. Many of these youth are suffering from mental and behavioral health conditions such as conduct disorder, oppositional defiant disorder, post-traumatic stress disorder (PTSD), depression, anxiety disorders, and

Investing in Children's Mental Health. Daniel Eisenberg and Ramesh Raghavan, Oxford University Press.
© Oxford University Press 2024. DOI: 10.1093/oso/9780190942014.003.0007

substance use disorders. Despite the mental health needs of this population, the majority of current juvenile justice services are more punitive than therapeutic, have little basis in the research evidence, and can even worsen antisocial behavior in some cases (Henggeler & Schoenwald, 2011). Examples of potentially harmful treatments include processing by the juvenile justice system (e.g., probation), transfers to adult criminal courts, surveillance, shock incarceration, and residential placements (e.g., boot camps, group homes, incarceration). Residential placements—which really refer to a location of care and not a type of treatment—are expensive. Because whether youth get better depends on the kinds of care they receive and not where they receive care, residential care has little evidence of effectiveness. Children with the severe problems typically treated by MST also do not usually do well in standard, community-based treatment.

MST, as its name implies, brings a systems-oriented approach to helping youth with severe mental health needs and their families. This approach takes the focus away from the child as the problem and addresses the ecosystem surrounding the child: the family, peers, school, and variety of services that need to be coordinated. This approach requires an intensive intervention that can manage the complexity of the system surrounding the child. Caseloads are limited to no more than six clients per therapist, allowing the therapist to have frequent contact with the child and family, and to be on call at all times to respond to crises or other emergent needs. The course of therapy is limited to three to six months, which introduces pressure to make fast progress and keeps costs under control.

MST is also notable for its intensive support of implementation and sustainment. MST Services provides comprehensive training for therapists and supervisors, as well as support to provider organizations to ensure they are prepared to deliver the program and can fund it sustainably. There are also multiple layers of quality monitoring and support, in coordination with the MST Institute and Network Partners.

Evidence of Effectiveness

MST has one of the strongest bases of evidence among all programs addressing children's mental health. It is one of just a few programs designated as Model Plus in the Blueprints registry, which requires multiple independent, rigorous replication studies by researchers other than the program developers. According to the summary in Blueprints, 25 evaluations of MST have been published, and 22 of these used randomized designs, the gold standard to assess treatment effectiveness. The majority of these studies were conducted with youth who had engaged in violent behaviors, substance abuse, or problematic sexual behaviors. Most of the randomized studies found that MST produces short- and long-term reductions in criminal behavior and residential or foster care placements. A recent meta-analysis concluded that MST has modest but long-lasting effects, with larger effect sizes for higher risk youth (Dopp et al., 2017). Another strength of MST's evidence is that it has shown positive outcomes across settings in several different countries and with a variety of racial/ethnic and gender groups. As Blueprints notes in its summary of MST, it has been found effective for both males and females and has also been shown to be equally effective with youth of different age and ethnic backgrounds.

MST Services compiles a comprehensive, annual summary of evidence, including every known evaluation study, available on their website (https://www.mstservices.com/). As of 2022 this summary lists 91 published evaluation studies, including 28 randomized trials, yielding more than 170 peer-reviewed articles. Most of the studies (64 of 91) are by independent researchers, not involving an MST developer. Overall, long-term rearrest rates in studies with youth who have engaged in illegal behaviors are reduced by a median of 42%. Residential or foster care placements, across all MST studies, are reduced by a median of 54%. Other positive outcomes include improved family functioning, decreased substance use among youth, fewer mental health problems for youth, higher levels of client satisfaction, and considerable cost savings. Some studies have included long-term follow-up and show long-lasting benefits. For example, a 22-year follow-up study by the Missouri Delinquency Project showed that youth who receive MST have 36% fewer felony arrests; 75% fewer violent felony arrests; 33% fewer days incarcerated; 37% fewer divorces, paternity, and child support suits; and 56% fewer felony arrests for siblings (Sawyer & Borduin, 2011). Finally, MST's theory of change has been supported by treatment process research: studies suggest that improving family relations is the key mechanism through which MST acts to reduce youth antisocial behavior.

Although MST is backed by an impressive base of research, there are still questions to resolve. As program developer Scott Henggeler noted to us, it is largely settled that MST produces good outcomes, so the focus has turned to implementation issues: In what type of contexts is MST most impactful, and what are the best ways to implement MST efficiently and sustainably? Research on these issues will continue to shed new light on the main puzzle raised by this chapter: Why is MST not reaching more youth and families who would benefit, and what can be done to increase its reach?

Costs: MST Is Expensive but Ends Up Saving Money

Experts estimate that MST is reaching fewer than 10% of high-risk youth who would benefit, such as those who have been arrested and are at risk for out-of-home placements (Henggeler & Schoenwald, 2011). More broadly, MST reaches only about 1% of youth with severe emotional disturbances (Bruns et al., 2016). An obvious barrier to wider dissemination is the cost of implementing and delivering the program. The per-participant cost is in the range of $7,000–$13,000, according to Blueprints. As one of the program developers, Charles Borduin, pointed out to us, the program appears expensive until one considers the alternatives. In the absence of MST, children are more likely to end up in expensive residential placements and to continue committing crimes, all of which represent significant economic burdens. Thus, the question becomes: How do the upfront costs of implementing and delivering MST compare with the avoided costs of placements and downstream consequences of inadequate or ineffective services?

The Washington State Institute for Public Policy (WSIPP) estimates a benefit–cost ratio of 1.77 (benefits of $14,134, costs of $7,973), with a 76% chance of positive net benefits (acknowledging the uncertainty surrounding the estimates). The majority of the economic benefits are from reduced crime, with additional benefits from employment-related earnings through increased high school graduation and reduced healthcare use. Their meta-analysis found small but lasting effects on crime and larger effects on behavioral problems. The uncertainty about the net benefits—a 76% chance is encouraging but far from certain—seems to be driven by the fact that the crime reductions are statistically significant at a strong but not definitive level. WSIPP does not include health-related quality of life improvements directly in the economic benefits, so the full benefits to society are likely to be even greater if they could be properly quantified. Also, their estimates do not account for reduced residential or foster care placements; these are often touted as the most immediate economic benefit of MST.

Indeed, other economic estimates indicate an even more favorable benefit–cost ratio. Dopp and colleagues (2014) estimated the long-term economic benefits of MST, based on the Missouri Delinquency Project trial. They focused on benefits stemming from reduced crime rates (recidivism) for both program participants and their siblings who were closest in age. Overall, they found a benefit–cost ratio of over 5 to 1. Although MST initially costs significantly more than the alternative in their analysis (individual therapy)—over $11,000 per participant, as compared with just over $2,000—these extra costs are recovered from a government budget perspective within a few years. The benefit–cost ratio becomes very favorable once the costs of crimes to victims are included. These estimates are still conservative in a couple important respects: They are comparing MST to individual therapy, which is more effective and less costly than the residential placements commonly used in many communities, and the analysis does not include other potential economic benefits, such as increased employment and earnings, which were not tracked in this study. The estimated economic benefits for siblings (nearly $8,000 per MST family) are also notable, because they represent a rare example of evidence for spillover benefits of a mental health intervention—that is, in which the benefits of the intervention extend beyond just the direct recipient of the services to, in this case, the recipient's sibling. This spillover benefit is consistent with the family-based and social-ecological approach of MST.

Although the overall economic returns for MST appear to be strong, this does not necessarily mean that funding MST will be attractive from the standpoint of specific government agencies or other decision-making organizations. There are steep challenges in aligning financial incentives; like many other programs for children and youth with complicated needs, MST suffers from the "wrong pockets" problem in which an organization investing in intensive services does not see much of the subsequent savings that result. Also, there are substantial costs outside of direct service delivery— most notably, support for implementation, quality, and fidelity— much of which occur early in the implementation process. There are also multiple payers with differing financial stakes, including Medicaid, private insurers, and the juvenile justice system.

Specifically, four funding issues are critical to address in policies that support evidence-based treatments like MST, according to Henggeler and Schoenwald (2011). First, if it is more profitable for a local provider organization to deliver a treatment of dubious effectiveness (such as residential treatment) to a specific target population than to deliver an evidence-based treatment for that population, odds are low that the evidence-based treatment will substantially penetrate that market of service providers. Second, where evidence exists that model-specific training and implementation support are needed to sustain treatment fidelity and associated client outcomes, funding must be provided for the training and ongoing implementation support. Third, funding must be adequate to subsume the start-up costs associated with staffing and initial training incurred before services can be delivered and billed. Fourth, an adequate fit is needed between the payment mechanism and the characteristics of the treatment.

Enhanced Medicaid reimbursement has been the most common financing strategy to date for MST. It has been successful in many states such as New Mexico. As part of its support for the implementation and sustainment of MST, MST Services provides considerable information and guidance regarding the use of Medicaid to finance the program.

Pay-for-success, also known as social impact bonds, has been touted as a new strategy to help fund the wider spread of MST. Dopp and colleagues (2019) evaluated the potential to finance MST with this approach, using the basic criteria proposed by Lantz and Iovan (Lantz & Iovan, 2017). They find that standard MST and some of its adaptations meet the criteria and are promising candidates. In particular, MST addresses problems of interest to the public sector, has a strong evidence base, is economically attractive to the public sector, has clearly defined and measurable outcomes that can be achieved within a reasonable time period, and can be implemented without significant administrative challenges.

Suzanne Kerns at the Center for Effective Interventions is leading a pay-for-success initiative in Colorado to deliver MST in rural, underserved areas. This initiative arose from a call by the state government for innovation related to foster care children and children in contact with juvenile justice. Their project has $2.2 million in funding, with half raised from social investors as part of the pay-for-success model. This is the first pay-for-success project in the state, and one of the first anywhere to fund MST. Kerns notes that it has been considerable work to pull together, but she is optimistic this approach can become more efficient over time.

Other Implementation Challenges

The barriers to the wider reach of MST extend well beyond cost considerations. The program also contends with interests and attitudes that are firmly entrenched in the juvenile justice and child welfare systems. To illustrate this point, the program developer Charles Borduin shared an anecdote with us from a presentation he made many years ago to state administrators in Ohio. During his talk he noticed two men sitting quietly in the back of the room, observing his talk. After the talk he found out they represented residential treatment centers and were there to learn about potential threats to their interests. Borduin also shared an experience where he gave a talk as part of a videoconference series for juvenile judges. He listened to the next talk in the series a couple weeks later and heard the speaker talk about evidence in favor of residential treatments. Afterward he asked the speaker for the supporting references and was given studies that concluded the opposite. When asked about this, the speaker simply acknowledged to Borduin that maybe he should have read those reports more carefully!

Some of the providers we interviewed also highlight the entrenched attitudes and beliefs among judges, child welfare referees, and even families themselves. The traditional notion is that the child who is getting into trouble is the problem, and the solution is to send the child where he or she can no longer engage in the same behaviors and might be able to reform. This attitude turns a blind eye to the more complicated and challenging reality that the problem to be fixed involves not only the child but also the surrounding system of family, peers, school, and services. Providers also mention that MST is an uncomfortable fit for some therapists.

It is more intensive than most other therapies, and it focuses less on establishing a warm rapport with the child and more on functional improvements in the full system of support and risks. For some therapists, this might feel less rewarding and lead to burnout, even if the behavioral outcomes are better.

Another implementation challenge is how to fit MST with lower resourced, less populated areas. In a rural area with low population density, it is hard to maintain the intensive and frequent in-person contacts required by MST with a full roster of client families. Alex Dopp, an implementation researcher who has evaluated MST extensively, suggests that rural areas might require some combination of two strategies, both of which would require new flexibility in the MST delivery model: (1) blended MST teams, which are trained to deliver not only MST but also other evidence-based practices; (2) technology-based communication to replace some of the in-person contacts with clients and within MST teams (e.g., coordination, supervision). The latter has started to occur as a result of COVID-19 pandemic, which has forced many organizations to deliver MST virtually, as we discuss later in this chapter.

Lessons from Michigan and New Mexico

A number of states and communities offer informative examples of successes and challenges in implementing MST. One example is in Wayne County, which includes Detroit and is the most populous county in Michigan. The Guidance Center is a mental health service agency that has been providing MST to poverty-stricken areas throughout the county since 2013. We met with their MST supervisors and therapists, along with Kim Hinton, the Assistant Director of the organization, in their basement conference room on a cold spring day in 2019.

They have solved the funding challenge by working out a contract with Bridgeway, a care management organization that is responsible for coordinating the services for youth in the juvenile justice system. Based on estimated savings from reduced juvenile justice services (in particular, fewer costly residential placements), Bridgeway pays the Guidance Center a per diem fee to help support MST services. This fee is on top of Medicaid and other insurance reimbursements; this supplement is crucial because Medicaid has a relatively low reimbursement rate for this service and a high administrative burden.

The Center's team of supervisors and therapists believes that MST is having a positive impact in large part because of its focus on fidelity and outcome monitoring. They hear frequently from other professionals that MST is the first therapy they have seen that actually does exactly what it says it is going to do. They find the continuous consultation and support from MST Services to be highly valuable, and they also have ongoing professional development plans for therapists and supervisors, which keeps them working toward greater skill levels and higher fidelity. They also find the outcome data powerful and motivating for internal purposes and for communicating with other stakeholders in the county; MST provides a standardized platform for collecting data on outcomes such as staying in the community (avoiding placements), prosocial activities, school attendance, and arrest recidivism.

The team can easily rattle off examples of successful outcomes with clients, such as a boy who broke free from a life with a gang and drugs, and a girl whose family started to believe in her when she finally tested clean for drugs after a course of MST treatment. At the same time, they emphasize that in the vast majority of cases, it is simply not realistic to bring a family and child to an ideal state, because they are starting in such challenging and complicated situations. Small but meaningful successes are much more common. The team members also lament that potential success stories are often cut short by harsh decisions by judges and referees. For example, a child could be making great progress on nearly every front, but if he or she fails a drug test, that will often lead to an immediate placement and termination of MST.

The Guidance Center is hoping to expand to additional MST teams in the future, but the limiting factor at the moment is the modest number of referrals. Many fewer children are referred than the number of them who would benefit significantly. It is largely up to the juvenile justice system and the care management organizations in Wayne County to make the referrals. The Guidance Center is in regular contact with these stakeholders to encourage the use of MST rather than placements, but an entrenched sense of hopelessness and pessimism often favors the latter.

At a statewide level, MST experts point to the Southwest Family Guidance Center & Institute in New Mexico as one of the program's greatest success stories. Southwest Family Guidance Center maintains service delivery hubs in most of the state's largest cities, including Albuquerque, Santa Fe, and Las Cruces. The organization started delivering MST in 2006 and has expanded to cover much of the state with 11 MST teams as of 2020. Although they were not the first organization to deliver MST in New Mexico, they deliver approximately 80% of the program's services in the state. Some of the other main providers were greatly affected by a situation in 2013 where the state's Human Services Department cut off Medicaid payments after an outside audit claimed to find evidence of fraud; although this situation was not specific to MST, it affected the solvency of other providers who were delivering MST at the time.

The organization's leaders attribute their success in expanding MST delivery to several factors. First, they were able to secure support from the state government, which explicitly incorporated MST into its Medicaid program. Relatedly, they have benefited from strong preexisting relationships with the state's Children, Youth & Families Department (CYFD), the juvenile justice system, and other stakeholders. Next, they have been able to document a range of positive outcomes resulting from the program, including clinical symptoms, functional outcomes, and cost savings. Their outcome measurement has been bolstered by state contracts with the University of New Mexico to collect and summarize data routinely. Based on these data and the everyday experiences of the providers and families, they have developed a reputation for delivering MST with high quality and fidelity. The attention to quality and fidelity reflects the background of the organization's chief executive officer, Craig Pierce, a clinician who previously developed a strong appreciation for the importance of fidelity while delivering the program himself. He also credits the quality assurance and support from the Network Partner organization, the Center for Effective Interventions (led by Suzanne Kerns in Colorado, mentioned earlier). Pierce and his team embrace that support and believe it is essential to continue indefinitely.

In addition, the Southwest Family Guidance Center has had relatively low turnover and a strong organizational culture, which buffers against the stressful and intensive nature of delivering the program. They have typically hired their MST supervisors from within their teams of MST therapists, to ensure they understand how to deliver the program, and they have prioritized strong leadership and networking skills to facilitate strong relationships with other partner organizations in the state. Renée LaVail, the Center's clinical director, has been with the organization for over 12 years and corroborates that they have a supportive environment that prioritizes professional development and growth.

Both Pierce and LaVail acknowledge challenges and opportunities for even greater impact in their statewide work with MST. They would like to be able to reach more families, though not at the expense of quality and sustainability. It is particularly difficult to reach families in more rural counties, as noted earlier in this chapter. There has been a general push at the state level for using more paraprofessionals in mental health services, but it is not clear how that would help a highly specialized and intensive program like MST. They are also interested in incorporating telehealth for rural areas.

By necessity during the COVID-19 pandemic, telehealth has in fact become an integral part of MST delivery in all areas of New Mexico, rural and otherwise (and many other communities nationwide). LaVail believes that virtual communication will likely remain an important part of MST in many communities even after the pandemic subsides. She reports they are getting good outcomes thus far with telehealth adaptations of MST. Most of the communication with therapists and client families is through videoconference, although it is closer to a 50/50 mix of video and phone in some rural areas. Clinics have been able to expand their reach to additional rural counties in New Mexico. The Center for Effective Interventions, mentioned earlier, brought together supervisors across regions, and in collaboration they were able to solve problems adapting to the pandemic.

Beyond MST: A Focus on Practices, Not Just Programs?

Recall that in Chapter 5 we described an emerging debate regarding the pros and cons of structured social-emotional learning (SEL) programs versus "kernel" approaches. There is a somewhat parallel debate in the context of programs like MST that support youth in the juvenile justice system. Mark Lipsey has developed an alternative approach to interventions for these youth, the Standard Program Evaluation Protocol (SPEP) scheme (Lipsey, 2018). The idea is to identify generic practices that are consistently correlated with positive outcomes in meta-analyses, deploy a system for rigorously monitoring fidelity to these practices, and validate that such adherence is associated with positive outcomes. Lipsey (2020) points out that programs such as MST and functional family therapy (FFT) have achieved impressive penetration in some states, but, as noted earlier in this chapter, nationwide fewer than 10% of youth in juvenile justice are receiving these "model programs." Thus, alternative strategies are needed to identify and deploy effective practices. Elliott and colleagues (2020) and Lipsey (2020) offer a lively debate on the strengths and weaknesses of a focus on evidence-based *programs* versus evidence-based *practices*. In brief, this is a debate over whether we should focus more on standardized programs with strong evidence from randomized trials, such as MST and FFT, or the specific practices that appear to drive the beneficial effects of effective programs. The latter can be more flexibly implemented and are potentially more efficient but generally have less clear-cut evidence.

Equity Considerations

Like the programs featured in previous chapters, MST has clear potential to improve equity in children's health and well-being in our communities and is already helping to do so. It is specifically designed for youth and families who are at risk of entering the juvenile justice system, who tend to be disadvantaged socially and economically. As noted earlier, MST has shown beneficial outcomes across genders and racial/ethnic groups and has been implemented and tested in many countries beyond the United States for that matter. For communities that want to prioritize both cost-effectiveness and equity, MST clearly warrants consideration. Because MST is explicitly designed to respond to the specific needs and assets within a child's social context, it is well positioned to account for cultural and other family-specific factors.

Summary

MST illustrates a strong investment that reaches many children and yet could have an even greater impact with higher penetration throughout the United States. It has an impressive evidence base supporting its effectiveness and cost-effectiveness across a range of contexts, and the main question now is how to implement and sustain it on a larger scale. The key barriers to overcome include the coordination of financial incentives and resistance from entrenched interests in the juvenile justice and child welfare systems.

References

Bruns, E. J., Kerns, S. E., Pullmann, M. D., Hensley, S. W., Lutterman, T., & Hoagwood, K. E. (2016). Research, data, and evidence-based treatment use in state behavioral health systems, 2001–2012. *Psychiatric Services*, *67*(5), 496–503.

Dopp, A. R., Borduin, C. M., Wagner, D. V., & Sawyer, A. M. (2014). The economic impact of multisystemic therapy through midlife: A cost–benefit analysis with serious juvenile offenders and their siblings. *Journal of Consulting and Clinical Psychology*, *82*(4), 694–705.

Dopp, A. R., Borduin, C. M., White II, M. H., & Kuppens, S. (2017). Family-based treatments for serious juvenile offenders: A multilevel meta-analysis. *Journal of Consulting and Clinical Psychology*, *85*(4), 335–354.

Dopp, A. R., Perrine, C. M., Iovan, S., & Lantz, P. M. (2019). The potential of pay-for-success as a financing strategy for evidence-based practices: An illustration with multisystemic therapy. *Administration and Policy in Mental Health and Mental Health Services Research*, *46*(5), 629–635.

Elliott, D. S., Buckley, P. R., Gottfredson, D. C., Hawkins, J. D., & Tolan, P. H. (2020). Evidence-based juvenile justice programs and practices: A critical review. *Criminology & Public Policy*, *19*(4), 1305–1328.

Henggeler, S. W., & Schoenwald, S. K. (2011). Evidence-based interventions for juvenile offenders and juvenile justice policies that support them. *Social Policy Report*, *25*(1), 1–28.

Lantz, P., & Iovan, S. (2017, December 12). When does pay-for-success make sense? *Stanford Social Innovation Review*. https://doi.org/10.48558/5VZB-QF94

Lipsey, M. W. (2018). Effective use of the large body of research on the effectiveness of programs for juvenile offenders and the failure of the model programs approach. *Criminology & Public Policy*, *17*(1), 189–198.

Lipsey, M. W. (2020). Revisited: Effective use of the large body of research on the effectiveness of programs for juvenile offenders and the failure of the model programs approach. *Criminology & Public Policy, 19*(4), 1329–1345.

Sawyer, A. M., & Borduin, C. M. (2011). Effects of multisystemic therapy through midlife: A 21.9-year follow-up to a randomized clinical trial with serious and violent juvenile offenders. *Journal of Consulting and Clinical Psychology, 79*(5), 643–652.

7

Communities That Care

The case studies that we have examined thus far are focused on specific intervention programs and the evidence behind their effectiveness. But once an intervention is identified as worth delivering by a community or organization, how should they create an environment in which the delivery of those programs can flourish? And what are some evidence-based models to support and sustain the delivery of interventions in the community? Improving children's mental health is not solely a matter of selecting the right interventions; rather, decision makers need to consider the context within which these interventions are to be delivered.

Consider a gardening analogy. Growing a garden is not simply a matter of purchasing high quality seeds; it also demands soil preparation and maintenance. Even the best seeds cannot grow in poor soil, and similarly even the best interventions cannot take root if the ecosystem is underdeveloped.

Communities That Care (CTC) is a framework specifically designed to undertake the kind of soil preparation and maintenance that is necessary for interventions to take root and flourish over a long period of time. CTC is not a specific intervention or program, but a *system* that builds the capacity of communities to address adolescent health and behavior problems. In this chapter we examine a successful example of CTC and then consider its strengths and limitations from a broader perspective.

Investing in Children's Mental Health. Daniel Eisenberg and Ramesh Raghavan, Oxford University Press.
© Oxford University Press 2024. DOI: 10.1093/oso/9780190942014.003.0008

CTC in Franklin County and North Quabbin

In the fall of 2020, the COVID epidemic was still raging across the United States. In the bucolic area of Franklin County and the North Quabbin in Massachusetts, this meant that the meeting of the local CTC coalition had to be conducted online via videoconference. One of the CTC co-coordinators, Kat Allen, opened the meeting with a warm welcome. The group on the call was informal in many ways—for example, one participant was seen on the screen with her small dog, who sat with the seasoned air of one who has been there many times before. As in other meetings we attended with this group, the meeting began with a fun or thought-provoking icebreaker that allows participants to share a bit about themselves personally or their perspective on their work. These icebreakers cover everything from what each person appreciates most about the community, to favorite Halloween costumes people have worn, to interesting experiences with haircuts during the pandemic. This informal approach balances nicely with the clear professionalism and dedication of the group.

The coalition has been in operation continuously since 2003. Kat Allen stepped in as the coalition coordinator in 2004, and her colleague Rachel Stoler joined as co-coordinator in 2016, having been intimately involved in the coalition since its inception. Thus, the coalition has had steady leadership throughout its history. The coalition began in this region of Massachusetts in large part because the purveyor organization of CTC at the time, Channing Bete, happened to be located within Franklin County in Deerfield. They had an interest in implementing CTC locally, so they asked around about what would be the right agency, and they offered it at a reduced price. They found Community Action Pioneer Valley, the region's anti-poverty organization, to coordinate the coalition, and a local lumberyard owner stepped up and picked up the rest of the cost. Meanwhile, the Franklin Regional Council of Governments— the region's substitute for a county government, which no longer exists in Massachusetts—had received funding from the Substance Abuse and Mental Health Services Administration (SAMHSA) through the Drug-Free Communities program, which similarly emphasizes community building and using data. These funds permitted the Franklin Regional Council of Governments and Community Action Pioneer Valley to become cohosts of the initiative. Thus, the coalition started as a partnership between the business community, the nonprofit sector, and local government.

The culture of the Franklin County and North Quabbin Region, located in rural Western Massachusetts, is generally viewed as collaborative, and the coalition has strived to leverage and enhance that strength. Since its inception, the coalition has worked on a variety of projects focused on improving the lives of adolescents in the region. It worked with schools to set up a Teen Health Survey in 2003 with five local districts, and they soon expanded the survey to all nine districts in the region. The initial surveys showed high rates of youth substance use, especially marijuana and alcohol. The surveys also illuminated key risk and protective factors. The coalition decided to focus on three of these factors: family management practices (e.g., clear rules, monitoring, and awareness), parental attitudes toward youth substance use, and community laws and norms toward youth substance use. They formed work groups around these priority factors, as well as a regional school health task force. In later years they added two more priority risk factors based on changes in the data: perception of risk of harm from youth substance use, and symptoms of depression and anxiety, which were especially apparent among girls in the survey data. They also added a youth leadership board and a racial justice work group.

By nearly every measure, the results of the coalition's work have been impressive, based on their community surveys over the years. Since 2003 the prevalence of alcohol use, cigarette use, and marijuana use among adolescents in the county has fallen by more than 80%, 85%, and 60%, respectively. These declines are considerably larger than national trends during this period. The priority risk factors have similarly declined substantially—particularly family management problems and family attachment.

The work necessitates nimbleness and willingness to change direction in pursuit of what works. For example, in their early years the coalition was promoting evidence-based parent education programs (such as Guiding Good Choices) through training of trainers and mini-grants in an effort to change parental attitudes related to substance use. But recruiting parents to attend was a perennial challenge, and after finding little progress in this risk factor in 2006 and 2009, the coalition implemented a social norms marketing program with a focus on those attitudes and behaviors. An intensive communications effort was launched: They worked with schools to send postcards home, and they worked with businesses to get messages on pizza boxes, grocery bags, paper napkins, fortune cookie messages, windows, banners, billboards, and the radio.

Based on outside research they came across, they promoted family dinners as one of the key practices. This fit well with the emergent context at the time—efforts to reduce childhood obesity and the economic recession in which families were trying to save money by making their own meals at home more often. Funding sources were drying up for a specific focus on substance use, and new state funding was available to address nutrition and physical activity. They found an 11% increase in youth having dinners with their family, and for the first time they also found a significant improvement in parental attitudes and behaviors related to youth substance use.

The Franklin County and North Quabbin CTC coalition has been featured in the *Stanford Social Innovation Review* as an example of how an organization can achieve collective impact through an emphasis on emergent rather than predetermined solutions (Kania & Kramer, 2013). The idea is that the best solutions to complex community-level problems cannot necessarily be known in advance; this goes beyond the traditional approach of assessing needs, selecting a strategy, and then evaluating the impacts retrospectively. Rather, a collective impact approach can identify emergent solutions by focusing on shared goals, measuring and sharing data frequently, and implementing new solutions based on the data and other opportunities that arise over time.

The coalition brings together stakeholders from a diverse set of local organizations and interests. These include schools, the Big Brothers Big Sisters organization, housing assistance organizations, the district attorney's office, the community health improvement plan (CHIP), a local opioid task force, and other youth-serving and family-serving organizations. At a meeting we attended, when they discussed another potentially competing group that was not already involved in their coalition, they focused on opportunities for including that group in upcoming events and meetings. At another meeting, some of the attendees persistently asked a series of provocative and important questions related to racism, and the leaders of the coalition responded with thoughtful and appreciative answers. The inclusive and collaborative culture appears to welcome, rather than deflect or resist, difficult questions and potentially competing groups and ideas.

The coalition aims to connect and amplify available resources in the community, more so than produce a new set of resources. This approach is more sustainable for their group of mostly volunteer participants, and it lends itself to strong partnerships. In fact, Kat Allen identified "synergy" and "amplification" as the two words that best capture their strengths and successes. For example, during a meeting in fall of 2020 the group discussed expanding their work related to the parenting guide they produce each fall, such as offering presentations on the topics in the guide. Kat suggested, to keep the workload reasonable, that they focus on promoting existing presentations and resources from local advocacy and service organizations. That suggestion then led to the idea for their group to host a public radio and television show where they can interview and feature local authors from the parent guide.

Collective impact work also requires that decisions be data driven. Consequently, the coalition has a consistent focus on data and measurement, which are evident in all the meetings we attended. One meeting included a brief presentation of the 2020 student health survey, which has been conducted every year since 2003. Participation in the survey was slightly lower than usual due to the school shutdowns from the COVID pandemic, but still high by general standards of survey research: 85% for 8th graders, 75% for 10th graders, and 58% for 12th graders. The survey focused on measuring school climate (using the U.S. Department of Education's School Climate Survey), and the data covered areas such as "Engagement" (cultural, relationship, participation), "Safety," and "Environment," with "very favorable," "favorable," and "not favorable" ratings attached to each average score. For the most part the ratings were in the "favorable" range, illustrating the strengths of the community's and coalition's work but also the opportunity to continue improving. The presenter of the data, Sage Shea, the coalition's on-staff evaluator, noted some small negative changes in perceptions related to equity (although most students still had favorable views) and acknowledged this could either be a real change in what's happening or a change in norms and perceptions, or both. The discussion quickly turned to questions such as "How do we turn these insights into findings?" and "What are the root causes that could be addressed?" The group also discussed whether to modify their regular slate of surveys and add a new survey targeted to the current situation in the pandemic.

CTC on a National (and International) Scale

Franklin County is one of many communities where CTC has been used successfully. The program has a strong presence in many U.S. states and in several other countries including Australia, Chile, Colombia, Germany, Mexico, and Sweden. CTC was originally developed by J. David Hawkins and Richard F. Catalano, researchers at University of Washington. Its dissemination and implementation are now supported by the University of Washington's Center for Communities that Care, directed by Kevin Haggerty.

In contrast to other programs that we have discussed in this book, CTC is not about delivering a particular program or intervention with specific content to recipients. Instead, it is about providing a structure and process through which communities can uncover problems afflicting young people in their community, identify solutions (such as an evidence-based program or service), and then implement and evaluate those solutions. This happens using a defined 5-stage process. CTC provides a structure for engaging stakeholders, establishing a shared vision, assessing levels of risk and protection, prioritizing risk and protective factors, and setting measurable goals. CTC guides the community coalitions to choose tested, effective programs and to implement the programs with fidelity. CTC also assists community coalitions to monitor implementation and outcomes of those programs and make adjustments in programming if indicated by the data. It is installed in communities through a series of six training events delivered over the course of 6–12 months by certified CTC trainers.

There are several attractive features about a model such as this. CTCs are inherently bottom-up and rely on the superior understanding of local needs and ways to address them that only knowledgeable community members and organizations can provide. This is why a coalition is so important—getting a range of voices is key to harvesting this collective local knowledge and experience. Second, the role of trainers is more as consultants of the process; in this way CTC resembles a more formal business consulting role. CTC has a research partner, Bach Harrison, which helps develop, implement, and evaluate the surveys that a community coalition might not have the capacity to do by itself. CTC trainers also help communities weigh the evidence of the solutions that the coalition wishes to implement in its region by acting as non-conflicted consultants. But the choice of what to implement within the community remains the decision of the coalition. Finally, the design of CTC supports sustainment. Because the programs that address community needs are democratically determined within the coalition, coalition members are invested in ensuring that these programs persist at least until those needs are no longer present. As illustrated in our vignette of the Western Massachusetts CTC, local businesses are an untapped resource in local sustainment efforts, and the design of CTC offers a more grassroots approach to sustaining necessary programs.

The evidence of effectiveness and cost-effectiveness is generally strong for CTC. The benefit–cost ratio is estimated at approximately 5:1, according to an analysis by Washington State Institute for Public Policy (WSIPP), with similar results in articles published by the CTC researchers (Kuklinski et al., 2015). Those estimates rely primarily on outcomes from a multi-state randomized trial with long-term follow-up of the original cohorts, which has found sustained decreases in substance use, delinquent behavior, and violence through age 21 for the communities assigned to CTC (Oesterle et al., 2018). On the other hand, the evidence is weaker from an analysis of repeated cross sections from the same communities in that large randomized trial (Rhew et al., 2016). In addition, a quasi-experimental study of 100 communities in Pennsylvania found generally positive effects, more so for delinquency than for substance use (Feinberg et al., 2010). A more recent study in Pennsylvania found positive results for not only delinquency but also substance use and depression (Chilenski et al., 2019). Finally, there is some evidence that CTC is especially effective in communities with high poverty and other disadvantages (Brown et al., 2014).

In an interview with Kevin Haggerty and Shelley Logan, the Director and Operations Manager, respectively, of the University of Washington Center for CTC, they reflected that they know they have succeeded when communities start asking, "What is the evidence? Where is the evidence?" That mindset is central to CTC's approach in creating lasting changes in communities. Indeed, a sub-study of communities in the large randomized trial revealed a greater focus on evidence and prevention among leaders in CTC communities (Rhew et al., 2013). This shift in attitudes appears to be a key mediator explaining the positive outcomes for adolescents.

Like many other successful initiatives, CTC has continued to evolve over time. As a result of the COVID-19 pandemic, Haggerty and Logan's center has accelerated the development and availability of online training. This makes it possible to continue bringing CTC to new communities despite the pandemic, and it will make the program more widely accessible even after the pandemic. CTC has also increased its explicit focus on the Social Development Strategy (SDS), which has always been the underlying philosophy embedded in CTC. The SDS has also been central to more specific interventions that have shown long-term benefits for mental health and other outcomes, such as the Seattle Youth Development project and Raising Healthy Children.

The SDS has five main principles, each of which is important for achieving positive behavioral and health outcomes for youth (Haggerty & McCowan, 2018). These principles have parallels with the nurturing environments framework introduced in Chapter 2. First, a community should provide young people with developmentally appropriate *opportunities* for active participation and meaningful interaction with others. Second, it is important to teach young people the *skills* they need to succeed. Skills and opportunities must be carefully balanced, as too much skill without opportunities leads to boredom and too much opportunity without skills leads to frustration. Third, a community should provide consistent, specific praise and *recognition* for effort, improvement, and achievement. Fourth, a community should promote positive *bonding*—a sense of attachment, emotional connection, and commitment to the people and groups who provide that recognition. Bonding can occur with a family member, teacher, coach, employer, or neighbor. Fifth and finally, a community should promote *clear standards for behavior*.

COMMUNITIES THAT CARE   111

Through the process of bonding, young people become motivated
to live according to the healthy standards of the person or group
to whom they are bonded. Each of the five components of the SDS
appears to be a mediator of positive outcomes such as reduced substance use and reduced juvenile delinquency (Kim et al., 2016).
CTC also has parallels with process improvement strategies that
have been widely applied within both the private sector and government. The classic example of a process improvement strategy
is the Deming/Shewhart product design cycle of Plan-Do-Check-
Act, also known as Plan-Do-Study-Act (PDSA), which is an itera-
tive process to identify and implement process improvements. This
approach is now a recognized methodology in continuous quality
improvement (CQI) circles, having been successfully adopted
in healthcare and many other fields such as software development, environment management, student advising in a university,
manufacturing, trucking and freight operations, real estate, and
food service operations.

Finally, as noted previously, the CTC model has parallels with
collective impact, a concept that has gained popularity in the world
of social entrepreneurship and policy. Both CTC and collective impact emphasize building coalitions, merging interests and efforts,
evolving in response to continual monitoring of outcomes, and
driving changes through an organized infrastructure.

Equity Considerations

CTC has mainly been implemented and evaluated in rural regions like the community in Massachusetts that we profiled. These
communities tend to be less racially diverse than many urban areas
but are generally facing economic challenges and lower access to
specialized health programs and services. Thus, CTC has already
demonstrated an important role in addressing inequities across
urban–rural and socioeconomic lines. And although the racial/

112 INVESTING IN CHILDREN'S MENTAL HEALTH

ethnic diversity is modest in places like Franklin County and North Quabbin, that CTC coalition has shown a strong commitment to equity and inclusion across a variety of identities and backgrounds. It remains to be seen whether and how this approach can succeed in similar fashion in more populated and racially diverse regions, where building and maintaining all the essential partnerships across neighborhoods and organizations could be more challenging. One encouraging example is the city of Cincinnati, where there has been a long-standing, successful coalition to support children's health and well-being in the community. Although this initiative is not part of CTC (rather, it is now part of the All Children Thrive network), it shares many of the same goals and priorities, such as frequent measurement, evaluation, and adaptation by a collaborative and inclusive set of local partners.

Summary

Specific evidence-based interventions are not enough to support children's mental health on a community-wide scale. They are the seeds for would-be plants, and a fertile soil is also needed, in the form of a coalition of partner organizations working together to identify appropriate programs, measure their impact, and adapt strategies over time. CTC is a framework that provides this soil, and evidence to date generally suggests that it works. Researchers, policymakers, and other stakeholders will need to continue to pay close attention to ensuring that evidence-based programs have a suitable context in which they can flourish in each community.

References

Brown, E. C., Hawkins, J. D., Rhew, I. C., Shapiro, V. B., Abbott, R. D., Oesterle, S., Arthur, M. W., Briney, J. S., & Catalano, R. F. (2014). Prevention system mediation of Communities That Care effects on youth outcomes. *Prevention Science*, *15*(5), 623–632.

Chilenski, S. M., Frank, J., Summers, N., & Lew, D. (2019). Public health benefits 16 years after a statewide policy change: Communities That Care in Pennsylvania. *Prevention Science*, *20*(6), 947–958.

Feinberg, M. E., Jones, D., Greenberg, M. T., Osgood, D. W., & Bontempo, D. (2010). Effects of the Communities That Care model in Pennsylvania on change in adolescent risk and problem behaviors. *Prevention Science*, *11*(2), 163–171.

Haggerty, K. P., & McCowan, K. J. (2018). Using the social development strategy to unleash the power of prevention. *Journal of the Society for Social Work and Research*, *9*(4), 741–763.

Kania, J., & Kramer, M. (2013). Embracing emergence: How collective impact addresses complexity. *Stanford Social Innovation Review*. https://doi.org/ 10.48558/ZJY9-4D87

Kim, B. E., Gilman, A. B., Hill, K. G., & Hawkins, J. D. (2016). Examining protective factors against violence among high-risk youth: Findings from the Seattle Social Development Project. *Journal of Criminal Justice*, *45*, 19–25.

Kuklinski, M. R., Fagan, A. A., Hawkins, J. D., Briney, J. S., & Catalano, R. F. (2015). Benefit–cost analysis of a randomized evaluation of Communities That Care: Monetizing intervention effects on the initiation of delinquency and substance use through grade 12. *Journal of Experimental Criminology*, *11*(2), 165–192.

Oesterle, S., Kuklinski, M. R., Hawkins, J. D., Skinner, M. L., Guttmannova, K., & Rhew, I. C. (2018). Long-term effects of the Communities That Care trial on substance use, antisocial behavior, and violence through age 21 years. *American Journal of Public Health*, *108*(5), 659–665.

Rhew, I. C., Brown, E. C., Hawkins, J. D., & Briney, J. S. (2013). Sustained effects of the Communities That Care system on prevention service system transformation. *American Journal of Public Health*, *103*(3), 529–535.

Rhew, I. C., Hawkins, J. D., Murray, D. M., Fagan, A. A., Oesterle, S., Abbott, R. D., & Catalano, R. F. (2016). Evaluation of community-level effects of Communities That Care on adolescent drug use and delinquency using a repeated cross-sectional design. *Prevention Science*, *17*(2), 177–187.

8

Lessons Learned and
Remaining Questions

As we write these words, the world has been grappling for multiple years with the COVID-19 pandemic. The fear and unimaginable devastation worldwide have been slowly replaced with a hesitant return to normalcy in many places—a new normal where we have learned to live with new behaviors and practices. While human ingenuity and the collective actions of scientists, administrators, and members of the public are responsible for the success against the COVID-19 virus, the pandemic has laid bare some unpleasant truths. The World Health Organization reported that the world has seen a 25% increase in the prevalence of anxiety and depression (World Health Organization, 2022). The young have borne the brunt of this burden, with suicidal thoughts and self-harm increasing disproportionately among young people. At the same time, we have seen the limits of our health systems, as service delivery institutions have been stretched to their limits, and beyond.

If there ever was a time to invest in the emotional well-being of young people, it is now. If there ever was a time to invest in the practices, providers, and organizations that can help young people toward achieving mental health, it is now. This pandemic has brought to the fore the consequences of not having made these investments in the past and presents us with an opportunity to do so now.

What have we learned from the preceding case studies and our broader review of data, reports, and perspectives from experts and stakeholders? In this chapter we synthesize major themes, lessons,

Investing in Children's Mental Health. Daniel Eisenberg and Ramesh Raghavan, Oxford University Press.
© Oxford University Press 2024. DOI: 10.1093/oso/9780190942014.003.0009

and lingering questions. As would be expected for a complex topic such as children's mental health, there are as many new questions as there are clear answers. The discussion in this chapter sets the stage for a series of recommendations, organized by audience, which we offer in the next and final chapter.

Need for Better Evidence

One of the first lessons is that, despite the many important advances in knowledge over the past decades, we still need better evidence regarding the effectiveness and cost-effectiveness of programs and practices that can support children's mental health. As we saw in the case studies, even in heavily researched areas such as home visiting, parent training, and social-emotional learning (SEL), there are only a few programs that meet the standard for clear evidence of effectiveness, such as Blueprints' criteria for Model programs. And even those few programs have important lingering questions to resolve, such as the duration of effects or the translation of effects to various subgroups of young people.

There are many more programs in the next tier of evidence, the "promising" category. One reason for this is that there is not enough support for evaluations to move from good to great evidence, such as independent replication trials and longer follow-up. Research funding and scholarly incentives tend to focus on novelty, and not all registries make clear distinctions between levels of evidence. Scientific evidence is not a binary, "exists/does not exist" type of a construct; most pieces of evidence are only partial and have significant limitations.

Consequently, there is great value in investing in promising but unproven programs, as long as we rigorously evaluate the outcomes and thus reduce the uncertainty about the programs' effectiveness and cost-effectiveness. To take a simplified example, suppose we have program A that produces net annual benefits (benefits minus costs) of $1 million. We also have program B with uncertain benefits—a 50% chance of $0 net benefits and 50% chance of $2 million net benefits. If we take a conservative strategy of only investing in program A, we will derive $1 million in net benefits a year. But if program B has potentially higher effectiveness than program A, then there is a 50% chance that we are missing out on $1 million in additional benefits every year (assuming that program B actually has $2 million net benefits). In other words, we are losing potential returns because of our ignorance—not knowing about the potentially higher effectiveness of program B. Thus, our best investment strategy would include continuing to deliver program A, while simultaneously dedicating some resources to evaluating program B more conclusively. This evaluation research might be costly, but there is a reasonable chance that it will change our future investment strategies for the better and increase our future returns indefinitely. More generally, an optimal strategy is for some communities and organizations to focus on proven investments while others rigorously test new and promising ones.

Developing Public Health Interventions

When we analyze the gap between evidence and practice, we tend to look at programs with strong evidence and wonder why they are not being used more widely. We believe this approach is useful and underlies in large part our case studies and analysis more broadly. At the same time, however, it is also important to turn this line of thinking on its head: Start with the public health issues and context and ask whether and how we can generate evidence for programs that address those issues and context.

In fact, the world's response to the COVID-19 pandemic is a good example of this approach. Funding agencies have reoriented priorities, scientists and laboratories have retooled, collaborations across national boundaries have expanded, industry has mobilized, and vaccine development efforts have been channeled toward health systems of varying capacities (for example, whether or not they can sustain a cold chain for a vaccine). This is "public health–centered research" that starts with a public health problem and designs solutions accordingly.

What if we looked at the whole of children's mental health as a complex public health challenge and asked ourselves: What type of programs and services (whether in existence currently or not) would best meet that challenge, and how can we best deliver those programs and services? Although children's mental health is more complex in many respects than a specific virus, the basic idea remains valid—if we start with the public health challenge and its surrounding context, we are most likely to develop and implement effective solutions. This path is in fact how many of the successful programs in our case studies were started; the developers designed a program or service to meet a particular public health challenge and context.

What would this type of an enterprise look like? In his influential paper "Sick Individuals and Sick Populations," the late epidemiologist Geoffrey Rose outlined an important distinction (Rose, 1985). Medical treatments are typically designed to pull at the tails of a disease distribution. For example, if someone has a high severity of depression, we administer treatments to reduce the severity of illness. Other examples abound—we administer blood pressure medications to lower high levels of blood pressure, to take Rose's original example. But pulling at the tail of a disease does little to alter the distribution of disease in the population—in order to do that, we have to shift the entire distribution of the disease. This thinking means that we cannot treat our way to population health. All the lung specialists, and respiratory technicians, and ventilators, and oxygen canisters, and intensive care beds, and dedicated nurses will not arrest the progression of the COVID pandemic. We need preventive behaviors such as wearing masks and limiting social interactions, and we need vaccines.

If we are to extend this analogy to children's mental health, we need to emphasize the development of "social vaccines." This means coming up with interventions that are preventative rather than curative, that can be directed toward populations rather than at individual children, and that address the determinants of disease rather than the disease itself. Social vaccines address the social, economic, structural, and developmental determinants of mental health (Allen et al., 2014; Baum et al., 2009). The nurturing environments framework suggests that the most promising ways to address these determinants is by limiting toxic exposures, promoting and reinforcing prosocial behaviors, limiting opportunities for problematic behaviors, and promoting psychological flexibility (Biglan et al., 2012). Such interventions usually lie outside the medical-psychological treatment ecology. In this book, we have discussed examples of potential social vaccines, such as home visiting and parenting programs, that address the circumstances and contexts that promote healthy child nurturing. There are several others, and our intention in this book is to ensure that as we support and invest in treating the urgent needs of children, we do not ignore the upstream investments that can be made in assuring the well-being of children.

Standardized Programs, Adaptations, and Kernels

When we consider the relevance of a program to a particular community or population, there is always the question of whether and how to adapt the program to the local context. Can we safely expect that the standardized program, for which we already have evidence of effectiveness in other contexts, will be effective in this new context? Or do we need to make adjustments or even start over with a completely different approach?

In confronting this dilemma, the first step is to determine the core components or elements, often referred to as "active ingredients," that are essential for making an evidence-based program effective. For example, in the Nurse–Family Partnership the core elements include educating the mother about child health, nutrition, and safety, and role-modeling sensitive and supportive interactions with the child; and in multisystemic therapy (MST) they include the promotion of positive relationships with family members and reducing interactions with deviant peer groups. These core components exert their effects on outcomes (such as child behavior) through mediating factors (such as increasing mother–child attachment). These core components along with their mediators form the crux of the intervention, and understanding them in unison is to understand how a program works—the "science of how" (Raghavan et al., 2019). Chapter 8 of a recent consensus report by the National Academies (2019) offers approaches to the identification of these core elements through research on mediators of program effects as well as multifactorial study trial designs. Once the core components have been identified, ensuring that they are being delivered with high fidelity is key to assuring program effectiveness. This is why, for example, MST is delivered only with systematic tracking of quality and fidelity measures supported by MST Services.

Establishing core components thus lays the foundation for adaptations, scaling up, and continuing to improve programs and services (Ferber et al., 2019). If and when adaptations are necessary for a local context, an approach grounded in community-based participatory research (CBPR) is often helpful. This approach involves community stakeholders closely in the process of determining the best intervention approach and delivering it successfully. There are many levels of adaptation. The "surface structure" of the intervention can be adapted by changing its language (e.g., translating materials), changing who delivers the intervention (e.g., training peer facilitators, or providers of a particular gender), and by changing program materials (e.g., adapting treatment manuals, or changing videos to show families from varied racial backgrounds) (van Mourik et al., 2019). Further, "deep structure adaptations" can also be performed, with changes in specific content, or incorporating cultural elements and norms. Communities That Care (CTC) epitomizes the adaptation to local context, by galvanizing community members and organizations to determine priorities and deliver programs adapted for members of their community, as we saw in the case of Western Massachusetts.

A focus on core components has also led some people to ask whether communities and organizations should have more flexibility to deliver those components flexibly, in different combinations, rather than as part of larger, structured programs. This tension between fidelity and adaptation has played out for years; we briefly discussed this in the context of MST and strategies to support troubled youth in the juvenile justice system, as well as the contrast between the kernel approach and packaged SEL programs. In brief, our take on this issue is that, for the moment, structured programs like MST and Promoting Alternative Thinking Strategies (PATHS) generally have the stronger and deeper evidence base, but a modular approach is showing great promise in many contexts and will undoubtedly continue to evolve with richer evidence. Also, although not featured in this book, there are some examples of intervention strategies that blend some of the desirable characteristics of both the structured and modular approach. For example, the Modular Approach to Therapy for Children (MATCH) approach to therapy for children's mental health, developed by Bruce Chorpita and colleagues (2005), identifies core components of effective therapy and offers an algorithm for a personalized sequence of those components based on the child's needs and responses to the therapy.

In parallel with core elements of effective interventions, it is useful to reconsider core skills among frontline providers such as child therapists. Because research and training in evidence-based practices tend to pay more attention to what is common—rather than to what is different—between patients, a gap between insights gained through research and those gained through clinical experience exists. "Core skills" refers to a common set of skills that expert clinicians possess. Scholars have described core skills necessary for the effective practice of psychotherapy (Sperry, 2011); skills that have been described as core competencies include the role of trust, creative silence, relating, learning from experience, speaking, frame management, and incorporation of research-derived techniques, effective communications, safeguarding and promoting the welfare of the child, supporting transitions, working with and across multiple agencies, and sharing information. Investing in skills-based, in addition to content-based, training and ongoing supervision will go a long way in assuring that clinicians delivering services possess the capacity to successfully deliver such services in a manner that is useful to their clients.

Importance of Purveyor Organizations

Another clear theme in our analysis is the importance of organizations whose focus is to support the scaling up of specific evidence-based programs and services. These organizations are typically referred to as purveyor organizations or intermediary purveyor organizations. In each example of a successful program in our case studies, there was at least one purveyor organization that facilitated the program's dissemination, implementation, and sustainability, such as MST Services, PATHS Worldwide, and the Center for Communities That Care.

These types of organizations are generally well equipped to provide training and, in some cases, monitor fidelity and quality but often have less capacity and expertise to actively promote the wider reach of programs (Neuhoff et al., 2017). They frequently lack the entrepreneurial skills and resources to market the programs and extend their financial viability. A recent review by Proctor and colleagues (2019) identified 119 purveyor organizations supporting the delivery of 127 children's behavioral health treatments, which suggests a fairly mature industry supporting the deployment of mental health interventions.

It is clear that purveyor organizations are filling an important need in bridging evidence with practice. Service agencies can benefit from professional advice and support on a range of issues, such as the nature and needs of their clients and community members, their operational competencies in terms of being able to service this demand, their competitive advantage for these services within the catchment area, and their financial security resulting from this competitive advantage. In other words, they are seeking the types of services that consulting firms generally supply to businesses. In the mental health field, in contrast to much of the world of business consulting, community organizations can only find consulting and support from organizations with great expertise in delivering narrow solutions, not necessarily in solving broader problems.

In addition to purveyors narrowly focused on a specific evidence-based program, a broader type of purveyor organization can benefit the mental health field. Rather than support only a specific program, such an organization would assist an agency with an understanding of its clients and community and available programs and services in evidence-based registries. This organization could also help agencies make decisions to implement interventions based on formal assessments of needs, constraints, and opportunities. Agencies should be assisted with thinking about whether the offering of the services is in the best interests of the agency and its providers, what the appropriate mix of services is for its clients, and how this mix aligns with organizational competencies. Once decisions are made regarding service mix and organizational competencies, the purveyor organization would focus on agency operations, efficiencies in training, client assessment, intervention delivery, documentation, appropriate billing, and outcomes maximization, thereby strengthening the core mission of the agency.

Once programs are up and running, the broad purveyor organization could help the provider agency come up with a sustainability plan so that once grants and other initial funds are expended, the work of the provider agency does not come to an end. Although this type of broad support is still difficult to find, it is beginning to emerge in pockets. At a national level, the Substance Abuse and Mental Health Services Administration (SAMHSA) has developed the Mental Health Technology Transfer Center (MHTTC) Network, which supports a variety of organizations and networks with broader purveyor functions. In some respects, CTC is also an example of the infrastructure that can support communities broadly in the selection and implementation of evidence-based programs. It will be important to grow the funding base for these broader purveyor organizations; while purveyors focused on specific programs are typically funded in large part through revenue from delivering trainings, funding for broader purveyors will require different sources.

Importance of Local Champions and Leadership

The power of individual champions and leaders is evident throughout our case studies, starting with the program developers and purveyor organizations, and also in the communities that have successfully adopted and sustained the programs. For example, the PATHS program for SEL has made a positive impact on children in communities such as Cleveland in large part thanks to the persistence and spirit of everyone from program developers and purveyors to school administrators, principals, and teachers.

What could we do to make these champions even more numerous and more effective? One possible channel is by increasing the prominence of evidence-based practices in training programs for frontline providers, many of whom go on to become administrators and leaders in their service organizations. Preparing the mental health workforce to implement evidence-based practice has been highlighted as a priority in social work and other fields (Bertram & Kerns, 2018). In addition, effective champions must not only be advocates for particular programs and services but must also promote the rigorous use of data to inform needs and measure progress. They also need to engage the full range of stakeholders in the community. These principles are epitomized by the CTC coalition in Western Massachusetts, and Durham Family Connects, as we have seen earlier.

Financing the Implementation of Effective Programs

In all the case studies in previous chapters, financing has been and will continue to be a major challenge in scaling up the programs. Health services and programs are primarily funded through insurance programs in the United States, which are designed for individual treatment services. Financing for community-level, preventive programs is much less established. In addition, insurance and health funding in general tends to cover the direct delivery of services and programs but not necessarily the costs of activities that support the implementation of those services, such as training and fidelity monitoring.

As we noted in the chapter about CTC, we find it helpful to think of a gardening analogy, where programs and services are like seeds, and the implementation context is like the soil. The financing system is a fundamental aspect of the implementation context. Our current financing system involves paying almost exclusively for high-quality seeds with little attention to soil preparation— the context within which the services and programs are delivered. Over time, new programs will arise and old programs will fall away; the state of our science is always evolving. So being wedded to a particular program is not a good long-run strategy. What is needed is a well-resourced infrastructure that can continually assure good soil—that is, appropriately and sustainably deliver any program, whatever the state-of-the-art program might be at that point in time.

Although we are far from achieving this well-resourced infrastructure, we have one encouraging example from Medicaid—the Early and Periodic Screening, Diagnostic, and Treatment program (EPSDT). EPSDT is an investment in health surveillance, not in any specific treatment. Medicaid beneficiaries under the age of 21 years are entitled to a set of services—including physical examination and dental and vision screening—at an interval as determined by the state's Medicaid plan. Once any health problems are identified through such screening, the program supports diagnostic tests and supports treatment for those diagnosed conditions, even if those conditions were not covered originally by the state's Medicaid plan. Although EPSDT has not achieved universal reach for the intended population, it is more than halfway there; of the approximately 35 million eligible children who should receive an EPSDT screen, 21 million (59% of those eligible) received a health screen (Center for Medicare and Medicaid Services, 2019).

Role of New Technologies for Interventions and Scaling Up

Another recurrent theme in our case studies and the broader field of children's mental health is the rapidly evolving role of new technologies to deliver and support programs and services. The most obvious example is the increasing use of remote, virtual communications, which has surged by necessity during the COVID-19 pandemic. Even programs that had previously resisted the use of virtual interactions, such as MST, have adapted quickly, with apparent success in New Mexico and many other communities.

The Blueprints team did a survey in summer 2020 of their Model and Promising programs and found that more than half of them were already making much greater use of online tools (Blueprints for Healthy Youth Development, 2020). It will be interesting to see the extent to which these adaptations remain permanently in the aftermath of the pandemic. It will also be important to evaluate the relative effectiveness and cost-effectiveness of remote versus in-person training and other implementation support. As noted in the case of MST, this is a potential solution to the challenge of delivering the program in rural areas with low population density.

Broad Definition of Children's Mental Health

Collectively the case studies illustrate the importance of a broad, holistic definition of mental health. Across the gamut of programs such as home visiting, parent training, SEL, MST, and CTC, there are widespread efforts to improve children's lives through a wide variety of targets and developmental stages. What is the ultimate purpose toward which these investments are stepping stones? Is it merely the mitigation of disease, or can these investments have a broader purpose—that of supporting the flourishing of children, and their growth and development into healthy and happy adults? Children need much more than the absence of disease to flourish.

It can be helpful to consider a specific theory of child well-being, such as the two sources theory (Raghavan & Alexandrova, 2015). This theory posits that a child displays well-being by mastering developmentally appropriate capacities (reading, for example) that ensure a successful future for the child, given the constraints of the environment. Second, a child displays well-being by engaging with the world in what we might consider childlike ways (engaging in play, for example). Investing in treatments for child and adolescent behavioral disorders is not equivalent, and definitely not sufficient, to assuring their well-being.

Instead, ways to enhance the well-being of children must necessarily focus on the contexts in which they live, deploying a variety of interventions at the family or community levels to support the development of the child. Most of these interventions may even lie outside the health system and may have effects on a range of child outcomes. We have seen a number of examples in the U.S. context through our case studies. To take an example outside the U.S. context, consider India's school midday meal (MDM) program. The program began in 1925 as an attempt by a municipal corporation to increase school attendance in government schools and was adopted statewide by a few progressive states, until a 2001 Indian Supreme Court decision created an entitlement to a cooked midday meal to each child in a government or government-aided school in the country. Currently the largest school nutrition program in the world, the MDM program provides a hot cooked meal every school day to over 100 million children in over one million schools nationwide (Ramachandran, 2019). Evaluations suggest that the MDM has successfully eliminated classroom hunger and has advanced the goal of universal primary education. In addition, the MDM program has had myriad other effects upon the child and the child's household, such as improved academic performance (Chakraborty & Jayaraman, 2019), even though few would conceptualize feeding a child as an educational intervention.

Whether in India, the United States, or elsewhere, we need to continue to search for additional social interventions and innovations that respond to the local context and improve outcomes for children. These interventions and innovations are likely to be disruptive, having effects that were unanticipated by program developers. Creating community contexts and spaces for the emergence of these interventions, and ensuring widespread participation in their deployment—as is being done, for example, in the All Children Thrive movement (act-ca.org/)—may seed sustainable efforts at child well-being.

Assuring Equity in Children's Programs

The most cost-effective investments in children's mental health also have great potential to help address the vast inequities in our society across socioeconomic, racial/ethnic, and other lines. Among the programs that we profiled in case studies, each has been evaluated with a diverse range of populations and settings, and many are explicitly designed for families confronting significant challenges such as poverty or risk of entering the juvenile justice system. Some of the programs, such as Triple P and Durham Family Connects, offer a tiered system of support, with services in proportion to the apparent needs of the families. Programs such as Nurse–Family Partnership and Multisystemic Therapy are highly attentive to the home environment of the child and adapt their support to the specific needs of the families. When interventions are adapted in ways that make them more aligned with the culture of participants, they become more effective (Griner & Smith, 2006).

There remain many challenges to resolve, however, before programs and services for children's mental health can fully achieve their impact on improving equity in our society. Although the evidence for many programs has been collected with diverse populations and settings, we cannot assume that the evidence therefore generalizes to all populations and settings. Cultural considerations cannot be reduced simply to a handful of racial/ethnic categories, for example. There is a continual need for policymakers and communities to ask which programs and services are responsive to local populations' needs, and whether adaptations or different programs are needed in some cases. This is again a reminder of the importance of involving community organizations and members in the full process of identifying needs, and selecting and implementing potential solutions.

References

Allen, J., Balfour, R., Bell, R., & Marmot, M. (2014). Social determinants of health. *International Review of Psychiatry, 26*(4), 392–407.

Baum, F., Narayan, R., Sanders, D., Patel, V., & Quizhpe, A. (2009). Social vaccines to resist and change unhealthy social and economic structures: A useful metaphor for health promotion. *Health Promotion International, 24*(4), 428–433.

Bertram, R., & Kerns, S. E. (2018). Integrating evidence-based practice and implementation science into academic and field curricula. *Journal of Social Work Education, 54*(Suppl. 1), S1–S4.

Biglan, A., Flay, B. R., Embry, D. D., & Sandler, I. N. (2012). The critical role of nurturing environments for promoting human well-being. *American Psychologist, 67*(4), 257.

Blueprints for Healthy Youth Development. (2020). *Implementation during the COVID-19 pandemic of interventions rated by Blueprints as Model/Model Plus and Promising*. https://www.blueprintsprograms.org/implementation-during-the-covid-19-pandemic-of-interventions-rated-by-blueprints-as-model-model-plus-and-promising/

Center for Medicare and Medicaid Services. (2019). *Annual EPSDT Participation Report, Form CMS-416, Fiscal Year 2018*. Centers for Medicare and Medicaid Services. https://www.medicaid.gov/medicaid/benefits/early-and-periodic-screening-diagnostic-and-treatment/index.html

Chakraborty, T., & Jayaraman, R. (2019). School feeding and learning achievement: Evidence from India's midday meal program. *Journal of Development Economics, 139*, 249–265.

Chorpita, B. F., Daleiden, E. L., & Weisz, J. R. (2005). Modularity in the design and application of therapeutic interventions. *Applied and Preventive Psychology, 11*(3), 141–156.

Ferber, T., Wiggins, M. E., & Sileo, A. (2019). *Advancing the use of core components of effective programs*. The Forum for Youth Investment. https://forumfyi.org/knowledge-center/advancing-core-components/

Griner, D., & Smith, T. B. (2006). Culturally adapted mental health intervention: A meta-analytic review. *Psychotherapy, 43*(4), 531–548.

National Academies of Sciences, Engineering, and Medicine. (2019). *Fostering healthy mental, emotional, and behavioral development in children and youth: A national agenda*. National Academies Press.

Neuhoff, A., Loomis, E., & Ahmed, F. (2017). *What's standing in the way of the spread of evidence-based programs*. B. Group.

Proctor, E., Hooley, C., Morse, A., McCrary, S., Kim, H., & Kohl, P. L. (2019). Intermediary/purveyor organizations for evidence-based interventions in the US child mental health: Characteristics and implementation strategies. *Implementation Science, 14*(1), 1–14.

Raghavan, R., & Alexandrova, A. (2015). Toward a theory of child well-being. *Social Indicators Research, 121*(3), 887–902.

Raghavan, R., Munson, M. R., & Le, C. (2019). Toward an experimental therapeutics approach in human services research. *Psychiatric Services, 70*(12), 1130–1137.

Ramachandran, P. (2019). School mid-day meal programme in India: Past, present, and future. *The Indian Journal of Pediatrics, 86*(6), 542–547.

Rose, G. (1985). Sick individuals and sick populations. *International Journal of Epidemiology, 14*(1), 32–38.

Sperry, L. (2011). *Core competencies in counseling and psychotherapy: Becoming a highly competent and effective therapist*. Routledge.

van Mourik, K., Crone, M., de Wolff, M., & Reis, R. (2019). Parent training programs for ethnic minorities: A meta-analysis of adaptations and effects. *Prevention Science, 18*(1), 95–105.

World Health Organization. (2022). *Mental health and COVID-19: Early evidence of the pandemic's impact*. https://www.who.int/publications/i/item/WHO-2019-nCoV-Sci_Brief-Mental_health-2022.1

9

A Path toward Better Investments

In this chapter, we distill the lessons from our analysis into recommendations, organized by audience. We approach this task with humility. As we have seen in prior chapters, there is considerable uncertainty regarding many programs and services about their effectiveness and cost-effectiveness across the wide range of contexts in which they might be deployed. With these caveats, we offer the following map of a productive path forward based on what we know today.

Recommendations for Decision Makers

The first set of recommendations is for those who make decisions about how much and what to invest in children's mental health. These decision makers include public policymakers, leaders of health and social service organizations, and other community leaders.

Invest heavily in scaling up the delivery of high-quality, proven interventions. We have seen repeatedly in our analysis that the relatively small number of programs and services with the highest levels of evidence are still reaching only a small fraction of children and families who would benefit. There is a need to expand access to these interventions in order to enhance their reach. In some of the case studies we considered a variety of factors that are impeding greater reach of some of these programs. In practice settings that have the capacity to implement such high-quality interventions— which tend to be resource intensive—part of the solution may

Investing in Children's Mental Health. Daniel Eisenberg and Ramesh Raghavan, Oxford University Press.
© Oxford University Press 2024. DOI: 10.1093/oso/9780190942014.003.0010

simply be to place a greater emphasis on evidence of effectiveness for the investment of limited resources. This is beginning to happen more regularly, as, for example, in the Families First Preventive Services Act enacted by Congress in 2018, which ties investments in child welfare programs to programs with strong evidence of effectiveness. We need policies that support investments in children's mental health.

We want to be clear that this first recommendation is not advocating for a one-size-fits-all approach to children's mental health, or for a narrow funding mechanism that demands specific treatments, regardless of their appropriateness for a given child. In fact, as we saw in the case studies, many of the programs with the strongest evidence are those that explicitly account for and adapt to the social context in which a child lives, particularly their home environment and caregiver relationships. Denise Main, executive director of the Sunrise Family Center in Bennington, Vermont, spoke to us about how parenting interventions are challenging to deploy with a family that is, for example, housed in a motel and that presents with other more compelling needs such as food and stable shelter. Even as they emphasize scaling up programs with strong evidence, policymakers will need to appreciate the complexity of program delivery across diverse settings and prioritize programs that are best suited to the contexts of children's lives.

Invest in new and promising strategies as well and be flexible with the evidence. While it is important to invest in proven solutions, this cannot be the only approach. The problems and opportunities related to children's mental health are far broader and more complex than the limited set of proven solutions that are currently available. Thus, we need to continue to document and understand these complex societal problems and pursue creative new solutions accordingly. Discovery and implementation need to go hand in hand.

Consequently, decision makers need to have a flexible orientation to the support of evidence-based practices; they also need to invest in programs and services with promising but not (yet) definitive evidence, and that may perhaps be a better fit with the needs of clients, as long as there are provisions to collect rigorous evaluation data that will add to the evidence base.

In other words, we need to remember the old dictum that the absence of evidence is not the same as evidence of ineffectiveness. We need a tiered system of evidence-based policymaking and evaluation (Arnold Ventures, 2018). The ideal scenario, in settings where it is feasible, is for promising programs to be rolled out in an experimental or quasi-experimental manner, in which their outcomes are measured over time alongside outcomes from an appropriate comparison group (e.g., similar communities without the programs). This requires investments in data collection efforts within agencies themselves so that they can document their outcomes rigorously. It is not enough for frontline agencies to know that they are achieving good outcomes for their clients—they need to demonstrate that they are doing so in a transparent and replicable manner.

Invest in making evidence more accessible and useful. The past three decades have witnessed the rise of registries of evidence, designed as compendiums of evidence-based programs meant for public consumption. Some registries (such as the California Evidence-Based Clearinghouse for Child Welfare) are funded by state agencies, some (such as the Washington State Institute for Public Policy [WSIPP]) are funded by state legislatures, while others (such as the Department of Education's What Works Clearinghouse) are funded by federal agencies—all as a way to improve public decision making. Even independently run registries (such as Blueprints for Healthy Youth Development) have received some public funding. It is clear that there is a need for easily accessible sources of information required for public policy, and that many public agencies are putting their money where their needs are.

This is a trend that we strongly encourage. Academic researchers are incentivized to disseminate knowledge primarily to other academics, not to communities, service organizations, practitioners, and the general public. Policymakers and other leaders can serve to fund such a knowledge transfer and dissemination effort. This funding should support not only the development of information repositories but also the staffing necessary to provide ongoing support and expertise regarding how to use the registry information most effectively. A registry of evidence should not simply be a passive website or database; it is much more likely to be useful and engaging if it is supported by an active network of experts and peer users.

Our review of registries suggests that much of this work is unidirectional—providing an outlet for research evidence that was generated through the ideas and motivation of researchers and program developers. Because research agendas are primarily built around the interests of researchers and program developers, there is a risk that researchers will generate knowledge that is not always useful for communities and public policy. Reorienting the research enterprise toward usable knowledge should be a key function of registries, and one that, as yet, appears to be under-resourced. Policymakers and community leaders are in a position to offer valuable feedback to evidence registries (and by extension, researchers and program developers), such as pointing out gaps in the information and opportunities to make results more relevant and accessible. In some cases, this feedback process is already occurring, particularly in cases such as WSIPP where the institute serves as a legislative think tank and is directly connected to the state legislative process. This seems to us to be a valuable model, and such bidirectional exchange is critical to maintaining feedback loops that improve the well-being of our nation's youth.

Support the measurement of children's mental health at a population level. One of the barriers to greater and better investment in children's mental health is the lack of consistent measurement of needs and progress at the population level. In public health, surveillance is the systematic tracking of individuals with particular health conditions that then helps in monitoring new cases, quantifying caseloads, and evaluating the effects of treatments and policies. The United States actively conducts health surveillance at a national level for various conditions, particularly infectious diseases, through the National Notifiable Diseases Surveillance System. But when it comes to behavioral health, we compensate for the lack of surveillance through a patchwork of various other data collection mechanisms (Lyerla & Stroup, 2018). This includes surveys (such as the Youth Risk Behavior Surveillance System), sentinel event or condition registries (such as the National Incidence Study or the National Child Abuse and Neglect Data System), privately funded networks collecting aggregate data on defined indicators (such as Kids Count), or mortality data at the population level (such as the National Vital Statistics System, which contains information on persons for whom a behavioral health condition is a cause of death). While these data are useful for decision making, the United States lacks a comprehensive behavioral health surveillance system.

The Centers for Disease Control and Prevention has a Public Health Data Modernization Initiative that aims to create a disease surveillance architecture across the United States. Several other partners and stakeholders, such as the Council of State and Territorial Epidemiologists (www.cste.org), an association of epidemiologists working in state and local government, along with other groups are also at work on creating a surveillance architecture. These efforts have gained momentum now that the COVID-19 pandemic has highlighted the underdeveloped state of public health data in the country.

An extension of these efforts to measuring children's mental health would have several important benefits. These benefits include a shared understanding of needs to rally around, identification of specific and emerging priorities, and documentation of successes and failures. Additionally, incentives and rewards could be tied to making improvements in measures of children's mental health not just at an individual level, but also at a community level, fostering creativity, competition, and motivation to address this area. Developing a mechanism to assess the magnitude of behavioral health burden at a population level is critical to assuring the health of our nation's children.

Align incentives to improve children's mental health. Another major barrier to investing in children's mental health is the difficulty in aligning incentives. Incentives are well aligned if the department or agency making a financial investment also sees the returns to such an investment. However, in the area of children's mental health, the investors do not necessarily reap the rewards of their investment; this is sometimes called the "wrong pockets" problem. For example, multisystemic therapy (MST) generates high economic benefits relative to costs, but those benefits—such as avoided costs from residential placements and reduced costs from future crimes—are typically accrued by child welfare agencies and juvenile justice systems, respectively, not by the mental health agencies that deliver MST.

One solution to the aligning of incentives is to explicitly recognize this crossing of administrative silos and break those silos down. We might think of this as a structural solution to the problem. For example, the state of New Mexico locates its child protective, juvenile justice, behavioral health, and early childhood services all within a single Children, Youth, and Families Department. At a national level, the Government of Iceland's Ministry of Education and Children integrates education, sports, and children's rights within a single administrative umbrella. There is also the potential for financial solutions, where savings are estimated and shared across agencies, or administrative structures are repurposed to eliminate financial disincentives. The Urban Institute's pay-for-success financing proposal is one attempt at solving this problem directed primarily toward a governmental audience, while social impact partnerships or social impact bonds are another approach focused on constructing public–private partnerships. However policymakers go about solving the wrong pockets problem, it is necessary to ensure that agencies are incentivized to invest in cost-effective programs that improve the well-being of children.

Support the infrastructure for implementation of evidence-based practices. As we have previously described using an analogy of gardening, we need to tend not only to the evidence-based practices—the seeds—but also to the broader system and context that supports such practices—the soil. This system and context include how services and programs are organized and financed, and how community organizations and stakeholders work together. Purveyor organizations that support specific programs and services play an important role, as we saw in our case studies, and there is also a great need for intermediate organizations that have a broader scope not tied to specific programs and services. The role of decision makers here is key, since the regulatory framework and enabling policies are also central to successful implementation.

In 2018 the Substance Abuse and Mental Health Services Administration (SAMHSA) began the development of this type of broader infrastructure to support the implementation of evidence-based practices through its Technology Transfer Center Networks, with networks focused on Addiction, Mental Health, and Prevention. Policymakers and other leaders need to support the continued growth of this type of infrastructure. The National Child Traumatic Stress Network runs a nationwide initiative that has successfully led implementation of evidence-based treatments for trauma over the past few decades; many of these implementations involve policymakers in state and local government. The National Association of State Mental Health Program Directors Research Institute (since rebranded as NRI), was a pioneer in implementing mental health innovation in states nationwide. This focus still continues at NRI, such as their efforts at implementing electronic health records within public health systems. That implementation is context dependent has long been recognized by research funders, and the National Institute of Mental Health (NIMH) funds centers with an emphasis on implementation and sustainability under its Advanced Laboratories for Accelerating the Reach and Impact of Treatments for Youth and Adults with Mental Illness (ALACRITY) portfolio. Some of these centers have had longstanding collaborations between academia and government (e.g., the University of Pennsylvania and the city of Philadelphia), which have served as implementation partners.

Communities often face challenges in maintaining programs when the initial grant funding that supported the program ends. Consequently, supporting the implementation of evidence-based practices also means supporting their sustainment over time. Policymakers can do this in a variety of ways—some grants currently require sustainability plans, others offer dedicated resources for grantees to hire sustainability consultants, and a few offer resources for a dedicated team member focused on organizational health. Organizations can be incentivized to hire an implementation specialist, whose role can extend throughout the life span of the implementation process. However these arrangements are made, it is crucial that the delivery of effective programs does not come to an end when grant funding for the program does.

Engage with other decision makers in communities. The greatest success stories for children's mental health tend to occur in communities with a broad range of leaders working together. Policymakers and leaders of organizations must engage with each other as part of a coalition and movement focused on child well-being. For example, the All Children Thrive California initiative offers an innovative model for doing this, by engaging government leaders alongside service organizations, other community leaders, and parents and families in the community. There are also promising examples at the state level such as Minnesota and New Mexico as part of the Results First Initiative with Pew Charitable Trusts. The states took an inventory of their services and programs, assessed the corresponding evidence of effectiveness and cost-effectiveness, and came up with recommendations for improving the efficiency and effectiveness of their services. In a prior chapter we have discussed the role of Communities That Care, another example of how grassroots organizations can frame and drive an improvement agenda forward. Explicitly building the need for such grassroots involvement into state and local grantmaking is key to assuring their support.

Recommendations for Frontline Providers

The next set of recommendations is for frontline providers of services and programs for children's mental health. This includes teachers, mental health professionals, pediatricians and primary care providers, child welfare and social workers, and many others.

Support and help shape "practice-based evidence." In its earliest formulations, evidence-based practice was seen as a three-legged stool, with research evidence, clinical judgment, and consumer preference as its three legs. Those of you who are clinicians may be acutely aware of the limitations of research evidence: its sometimes-uncertain fit with the needs of the clients that you serve, the difficulty of finding relevant evidence at the time you need it, and the perceived devaluing of practice-based evidence at the altar of evidence-based practice. These are all valid concerns; the challenge is how to maximize the confidence that children are receiving services and programs that work, while also maximizing the value of providers' own experience and strengths.

As we have stated before, today's health environments require objective evidence of effectiveness. And skilled intervention researchers actively participate in the lives of frontline providers, studying topics such as the "usual care" (which can be surprisingly effective), implementation in frontline contexts, and ways to harvest practice-based evidence. Today's mental health landscape has changed considerably since Vijay Ganju's prescient description of clinician reactions to evidence-based practice two decades ago (Ganju, 2003). For these reasons, evidence-based practice should be viewed by frontline providers as a powerful decision support tool.

If frontline providers are active in the process for considering and selecting particular programs and services, they will likely be more motivated and empowered to ensure their successful implementation and sustainment. We believe that providers will benefit from familiarity with registries such as Blueprints, which can help lead to greater incorporation of core components of efficacious practice and discontinuation of program elements known to be ineffective or harmful. Providers also have an important role in helping to monitor and track client outcomes, which can lead to greater sustainment of evidence-based practices within local mental health organizations. Providers who view evidence in such an empowering way can easily become a champion for a specific program that fits especially well with their community's needs, or more broadly, a general advocate for the emphasis on evidence as a useful tool in the service of good client outcomes.

Insist on and support the rigorous evaluation of programs with promising evidence. The energy and support of frontline providers is also needed for communities to try programs with promising evidence and learn from the experience. Frontline clinicians may have knowledge of programs or practices that seem to produce excellent client outcomes but have not been subject to rigorous testing. In such cases, bringing such programs to the attention of decision makers and researchers is the only way for discovery to occur, and for the implementation of unstudied programs that may well prove to be more effective than the ones that we are widely deploying.

It is important that the metrics of success be improvement in child and family well-being, and that these outcomes are prespecified. There are several programs that can increase the number of clients served (a process measure) or demonstrate high client satisfaction. These are important considerations, but for the field to make true progress and ultimately improve children's mental health everyone must embrace a rigorous approach to evaluation of effectiveness.

This means measuring progress over time with more meaningful outcomes, such as mental health symptoms and risk, or broader measures of well-being and functioning, and using a credible comparison group, such as other clients and communities with similar preexisting risk profiles. Although randomized control trials sometimes raise concerns about fairness, they can be conducted in ways such that everyone in the study benefits, such as using an active control intervention or offering the program to the control group after a specified period. Many researchers are deploying pragmatic clinical trials, which are more naturalistic and better reflect what really happens in community mental health contexts, in close collaboration with providers. Frontline providers have an important role in supporting the evaluation science that will lead to this knowledge.

Embrace deimplementation and the need to change course as needed. Sometimes the interventions we deploy are ineffective or less effective than other available programs. These interventions may fit well with the program model, may make sense conceptually, and may be well liked by participants. But if the interventions do not produce desired treatment outcomes, they need to be jettisoned. Those of you who work in the field of substance abuse prevention are likely familiar with Drug Abuse Resistance Education (D.A.R.E.), a notoriously ineffective program that not only did not reduce drug use but, by providing information about drugs to impressionable children, also increased their curiosity about drugs and occasionally resulted in higher rates of drug use. D.A.R.E. was nevertheless widely deployed within school systems nationwide, a phenomenon that Ellen Barry, a *Boston Globe* correspondent writing about the program in 1999, explained as resulting from ". . . Americans' stubborn resistance to apply science to drug policy."

Cessation of ineffective programs is referred to as deimplementation. To persist in delivering an ineffective program is a waste of both the provider's as well as the participant's time. It diverts resources from other, more effective, activities. Sometimes, the intervention is actively dangerous, producing outcomes worse than doing nothing. Frontline providers need to encourage not only rigorous evaluation but also measurement of outcomes more generally. Any systematic initiative to track children's mental health at the community and population level will be meaningful only to the extent that frontline providers are involved and supportive. For example, in the Communities That Care (CTC) case in Western Massachusetts, we saw that the frontline professionals in the core of the community coalition embraced a successful change in direction for their initiative in response to community-level data showing a lack of progress. Even as providers focus on their essential day-to-day interactions with children and families, they must also embrace a broader emphasis on data and science to drive their community's investments of limited resources.

Support the continuum of implementation. Even after a community or agency has made a careful selection of an evidence-based program ("adoption"), the hard work has only just begun, as we have seen throughout this book. Frontline providers can do many things to support the successful implementation and long-term sustainment of programs and services. They can embrace the monitoring and support of fidelity to the core elements of the program by celebrating successes and viewing problems as opportunities for improvement in the interest of the children and families they serve. They can also help determine and refine adaptations of program features that are not core elements. In addition, they can help recruit more children and families in the programs, with the confidence that these programs are likely to be highly effective. Providers can also have an active role in seeking grants that will help the program survive, writing them in collaboration with grant specialists or academic partners, and in serving as ambassadors for the program in front of philanthropic and other funders.

Encourage peers to do all of the above. If there is going to be a movement on a grand scale toward more effective programs for children's mental health, frontline providers will have to be at its center. Providers have deep knowledge of their community members, the local conditions, and the programs they are delivering. They span two worlds—the world of the organization with its external priorities, and the world of the child and family with their internal lived experience. Many executive directors of mental health organizations are, or were, providers themselves. This boundary-spanning capacity, and their ability to speak to leadership, makes providers a unique resource in the investment enterprise. Each provider is in position to initiate improvements in the ways we have described above, and also to inform and motivate their fellow providers to do the same.

Recommendation for Researchers and Funders of Research

The next recommendations are for researchers and research funders focused on programs and services for children's mental health. This research area is inherently multidisciplinary and should involve a diverse mix of fields such as psychology, psychiatry, social work, public health, education, sociology, economics, and more. Funders include not only the various institutes within the National Institutes of Health but also the National Science Foundation, the Department of Education, and a variety of national and location foundations focused on health and social issues. As the number of extremely wealthy individuals and families continues to swell in the United States, private philanthropists also have an increasingly important opportunity to fund groundbreaking research that will advance children's mental health. Many of these philanthropists are motivated by personal connections to the topic of children's mental health. Given that mental health risks are perpetuated in large part by socioeconomic disadvantages, investing in children's mental health research is one of the best ways to help combat the ever-widening inequities in our society.

Fill in the gaps in evidence, particularly for preventive and community programs. While decision makers and frontline providers have much work ahead to support and implement investments in programs, researchers have an equally important task: to improve the evidence base. There are few programs with definitive evidence of effectiveness and cost-effectiveness, as we have discussed. The challenge of producing clear-cut evidence is especially difficult for preventive and community-level programs. Such programs are typically more complex both to deliver and to evaluate, as compared with treatments directed at individuals and families. Rather than shy away from these challenges and accept a lower standard of evidence, the research field needs to embrace the hard and complicated work to aspire to the same standards that are expected by individual treatments such as medications that undergo the FDA approval process. This means conducting large-scale trials with communities or organizations as the units of analysis, with follow-up periods extending multiple years and intermediate outcome measures to understand mechanisms of impacts. This type of study is expensive, which will require new commitments from research funders.

Resolve uncertainties around promising but unproven programs. While there are few programs that are definitively strong investments in children's mental health, there are many with promising, but not clear-cut, evidence. Researchers need to do more to resolve the uncertainties around these programs. Part of the problem is undoubtedly the incentive system that researchers face—they are rewarded mainly for innovative, groundbreaking work, whereas resolving uncertainties about promising evidence typically involves less glamorous studies that build upon or replicate previous trials. Therefore, leaders of universities and other research organizations can help by providing more explicit rewards for the practical and policy impact of research. Similarly, funders could invest more in large trials and replication studies that are needed to resolve whether promising programs truly work; the funding strategy of Arnold Ventures is a notable example in this regard, as mentioned earlier. A key aspect of credible replication studies is to involve researchers who are independent from the program developers and purveyors; such independent evaluation is one of the factors that distinguishes Model Plus from Model programs in Blueprints.

Distinguish core elements from adaptable features. Programs and services have the greatest potential for scaling up to reach large populations of children and families when they have clearly identified core elements, or active ingredients, as we saw in the context of multisystemic therapy (MST) and social-emotional learning (SEL) programs, for example. When the core elements are known, a program can be pared down efficiently to its most essential features, and it can be adapted to local contexts without sacrificing effectiveness. Distinguishing core elements requires research studies that analyze mediators of intervention effects and employ designs such as the Multiphase Optimization Strategy (MOST) framework (Gustaferro & Collins, 2019), which tests various combinations of program components in order to disentangle their separate impacts. In addition, identifying core elements open possibilities for investigating the benefits of modular approaches to delivering services, as in the kernels approach to SEL.

A focus on core elements is also consistent with the experimental therapeutics approach promoted by the National Institute for Mental Health (Insel, 2015). This approach requires first understanding which "targets," or mechanisms, an intervention engages; these targets can be cognitive, behavioral, emotional, or social. Second, once the intervention target has been engaged, the approach examines what happens once the intervention engages the target—the pathway that leads toward a change in the outcome. This approach has been used widely in the mental health intervention development, and in human services (Raghavan et al., 2019).

Increase the study of usual care, practice-based evidence, and treatment adaptation. The disconnect between how researchers see their work and how practitioners and communities view the results of such work is rarely apparent to most of us in academia. This disconnect grew so extreme that it took an act of Congress to support a new way of funding, conducting, and evaluating research, when it created the Patient-Centered Outcomes Research Institute (PCORI) in 2010. PCORI, however, is a modest and isolated solution to a wider cultural problem. Academic scientists need to find a way to overcome the powerful incentives built into academia, specifically for the types of research that lead to promotion and tenure and direct their expertise toward topics that frontline clinicians and consumer groups consider important. Funding agencies such as NIMH have seen a steady expansion of program-initiated research—funding topics that the agency or program believes are critical for scientific advance based on consultation with the leading scientists in the field. It will also be important to fund research that addresses the needs and perspectives of practitioners and administrators, which may not always align with the priorities of leading scientists.

Improve understanding of long-term consequences of childhood experiences. The intuitive appeal of investing in children's mental health is the potential for improving outcomes that endure through the many years of remaining life expectancy for young people. Researchers can help solidify this intuition with empirical data by investigating longitudinal associations between early-life mental health and outcomes in adulthood. There are very few large-scale epidemiological studies with mental health measures early in life and lifelong follow-up periods. There are a small number of well-known exceptions in the field, such as the Harvard Grant Study that tracked male undergraduates for 75 years, summarized in George Vaillant's books *Adaptation to Life* and *Aging Well*, and the British documentary *Up!* series that followed the lives of 14 schoolchildren for over five decades. Building on this work, we need larger and more diverse longitudinal studies of mental health following people for many years, if not decades. Such long-term studies cannot be conducted unless research funders invest for the long term. Most research grants fund projects that need to be completed within 2–5 years. Short-term funding is important because it allows funders to support a wider array of studies and interventions and then adapt funding strategies based on the results. Alongside short-term funding, however, funders should consider more long-term investments in longitudinal studies. Longitudinal studies can provide particularly rich information in areas that might not have been conceived of by its original researchers and can yield new insights into the dynamics of illness and wellness.

Recommendations for Families, Concerned Citizens, and Young People Themselves

Our final set of recommendations is for families, citizens who simply want to support the well-being and future of children, and young people themselves. We imagine this group includes you if you are reading this book. Regardless of whether you have a formal professional role that relates to children and mental health, you have an opportunity to make an impact.

Advocate for programs that have the best evidence. As voters and as members of communities large and small, you can encourage your policymakers, administrators, and frontline professionals to implement programs and services with the best possible evidence. You can start by informing yourself about the possibilities by browsing evidence registries such as Blueprints and talking with professional experts. Then you can ask your local administrators and leaders, such as school principals and leaders of youth organizations, how they are using evidence to select their programs and services and whether they might consider programs that you have identified through your search. And you can support and vote for the leaders who use evidence to guide their investments. A movement toward better investments can start not just with leaders and those with professional authority but also with the members of communities whom they ultimately serve.

Advocate for innovating with new programs and rigorously assessing the outcomes. You can also push forward the idea that gaining knowledge about the impacts of programs for children's mental health is a good investment. There are not enough programs and services with definitive evidence, so we need to learn as much as possible when we implement programs with promising evidence. Community members can help support a culture of innovation and learning, because when it comes to your community you—and not scientific researchers—are the experts. Your community has an opportunity to be on the leading edge of understanding how to invest in children's mental health.

Young people: Consider a career related to mental health. To young people specifically, we encourage you to consider a career path related to mental health. Educators and mentors, you can support young people in considering such a path. There are few areas with such broad relevance and significance; mental health affects nearly everyone and is connected to nearly every other economic and social factor of consequence. We hope this book has given you a better sense of how you might help improve mental health for children and other populations through a variety of career paths. You can work with individuals and families as a frontline professional such as a therapist or social worker, and you can also help address community-level and societal challenges and opportunities as a policymaker, administrator, entrepreneur, or researcher. There is no limit to the possibilities in the important work ahead, and you have a valuable role to play. We invite you to play that role.

References

Arnold Ventures. (2018). *How to solve U.S. social problems when most rigorous program evaluations find disappointing effects (part two - a proposed solution*. Straight Talk on Evidence, Issue. https://www.straighttalkonevidence. org/2018/04/13/how-to-solve-u-s-social-problems-when-most-rigorous-program-evaluations-find-disappointing-effects-part-two-a-proposed-solution/

Ganju, V. (2003). Implementation of evidence-based practices in state mental health systems: Implications for research and effectiveness studies. *Schizophrenia Bulletin, 29*(1), 125–131.

Gustaferro, K., & Collins, L. M. (2019). Achieving the goals of translational science in public health intervention research: The Multiphase Optimization Strategy (MOST). *American Journal of Public Health, 109*(Suppl. 2), S128–S129.

Insel, T. (2015). The NIMH experimental medicine initiative. *World Psychiatry, 14*(2), 151–153.

Lyerla, R., & Stroup, D. (2018). Toward a public health surveillance system for behavioral health. *Public Health Reports, 133*(4), 360–365.

Raghavan, R., Munson, M. R., & Le, C. (2019). Toward an experimental therapeutics approach in human services research. *Psychiatric Services, 70*(12), 1130–1137.

Index

For the benefit of digital users, indexed terms that span two pages (e.g., 52–53) may, on occasion, appear on only one of those pages.

access to care, 1
access to evidence, 133–34
adaptations, 118–21, 146
  deep structure, 119–20
  with new technologies, 126
  surface structure, 119–20
  telehealth, 98, 125
Adaptation to Life (Vaillant), 146–47
Administration for Children and
  Families (ACF)
  Home Visiting Evidence
    of Effectiveness
    (HomVEE), 40–41
  Title IV-E Prevention Services
    Clearinghouse, 25–26
adolescent mental health, 1–
  2, 9–10
Advanced Laboratories for
  Accelerating the Reach and
  Impact of Treatments for Youth
  and Adults with Mental Illness
  (ALACRITY), 137–38
advocacy, 147–48
Affordable Care Act, 41
African Americans, 50–51
Aging Well (Vaillant), 146–47
Ahrens, Jillian, 71–72
Aid to Families with Dependent
  Children (AFDC), 49
ALACRITY (Advanced Laboratories
  for Accelerating the Reach
  and Impact of Treatments for
  Youth and Adults with Mental
  Illness), 137–38

Aleardi, Joe, 82–83
All Children Thrive, 111–12, 127
All Children Thrive –
  California, 138–39
Allen, Kat, 103–4, 106
American Indians, 51
American Institutes for Research
  (AIR), 75–76
amplification, 106
anxiety disorders, 86–87, 114
Apache, 51
Appel, Heather, 37
Arnold Ventures, 144–45
Aspen Institute, 76–77
Australia, 107–8

Baron, Jon, 19–20
Barry, Ellen, 141
behavioral health conditions
  burden of disease, 2
  disruptive behavior
    disorders, 57–60
benefit–cost analysis, 10–11, 12–13
best investments
  definition of, 10–13, 16–17
  integrating frameworks for, 16–17
Bete, Channing, 103–4
Big Brothers Big Sisters, 106
blended teams, 94
Blueprints Programs for Healthy
  Youth Development, 3, 25–26
  criteria for Model programs, 25,
    115, 144–45
  funding, 133

Blueprints Programs for Healthy
    Youth Development (*cont.*)
  parenting programs, 62–63
  social-emotional learning (SEL)
    programs, 78
  survey of MST, 88
  survey of online tools, 126
bonding, 110–11
Borduin, Charles, 89–90, 93
Boston Globe, 141
Bridgeport, Connecticut, 82–83
Bridgespan Group, 28
Bridgeway, 94–95

California Evidence-Based
    Clearinghouse for Child
    Welfare, 133
CALM Program, 73–74
CARE (Cultivating Awareness and
    Resilience in Education), 73–74
career development, 148
Caring School Community, 78
CASEL (Collaborative for Academic,
    Social, and Emotional
    Learning), 70, 74–75
Catalano, Richard F., 107–8
CBPR (community-based
    participatory research), 119–20
Center for Communities that Care,
    107–8, 109–10, 121
Center for Effective Interventions,
    96–97, 98
Centers for Disease Control and
    Prevention (CDC)
  Community Preventive Services
    Task Force, 25–26
  Public Health Data Modernization
    Initiative, 135
CFL (Conditions for Learning)
    assessment, 75–76
champions, local, 123–24
Child FIRST, 42–43
children's mental health
  burden of disease, 2

current evidence and
    practice, 18–36
  definition of, 9–10, 126–27
  equity considerations, 128
  incentives to improve, 136–37
  investment in, 8–9
  long-term studies of, 146–47
  measurement of, 134–36
  recommendations for better
    investments, 131–49
  recommendations for decision
    makers, 131–39
  recommendations for families,
    concerned citizens, and young
    people themselves, 147–48
  recommendations for frontline
    providers, 139–43
  recommendations for researchers
    and funders of research, 143–47
  two sources theory of well-
    being, 126
  vulnerability, 1–2
Chile, 107–8
Chorpita, Bruce, 120
Cincinnati, Ohio, 111–12
Clark Elementary School (Cleveland,
    Ohio), 73–74
Cleveland Metropolitan School
    District, 123
  Clark Elementary School, 73–74
  Memorial Elementary
    School, 71–72
  Say Yes program, 76
  social-emotional learning (SEL),
    70–76, 83
Cochrane Collaborative, 26
Cochrane Library, 26
Cochrane Pregnancy and Childbirth
    group, 26
cognitive-behavioral therapy
    (CBT), 25–26
Collaborative for Academic, Social,
    and Emotional Learning
    (CASEL), 70, 74–75

Colombia, 107–8
Colorado, 92–93
Communities That Care (CTC),
    102–13, 138–39
  adaptations to local
    context, 119–20
  attractive features, 108–9
  benefit–cost ratio, 109
  cost-effectiveness, 109
  dissemination and
    implementation, 107–8
  equity considerations, 107, 111–12
  evidence of effectiveness, 109–10
  evolution over time, 110
  in Franklin County and North
    Quabbin (Massachusetts), 103–
    7, 123–24
  lessons learned, 141–42
  on national (and international)
    scale, 107–11
  Social Development Strategy
    (SDS), 110–11
Community Action Pioneer
    Valley, 103–4
community-based participatory
    research (CBPR), 119–20
community health improvement
    plan (CHIP), 106
community programs, 144
Conditions for Learning (CFL)
    assessment, 75–76
conduct disorder, 86–87
continuous quality improvement
    (CQI), 111
cost-effectiveness analysis, 10–11
Council of State and Territorial
    Epidemiologists, 135
COVID-19 pandemic
  home visits during, 39–40
  impact on children's mental
    health, 29
  impact on MST delivery, 94, 98
  impact on online training, 110

impact on Teen Health Survey, 107
  lessons learned, 114, 116–17, 135
CQI (continuous quality
    improvement), 111
Creating Resilience for Educators,
    Administrators, and Teachers
    (CREATE), 73–74
CTC (Communities That
    Care), 102–13
Cultivating Awareness and
    Resilience in Education
    (CARE), 73–74
cultural considerations, 128
current evidence, 18–36
current practices, 29–31

Daily News, 37
D.A.R.E. (Drug Abuse Resistance
    Education) program, 30, 141
decision makers
  engagement with, 138–39
  recommendations for, 131–39
deimplementation, 32–33, 141–42
Deming, David, 77
depression, 86–87, 114
Detroit, Michigan, 94
developmental perspective, 15
Dinkins, Maria, 72
disruptive behavior disorders, 57–60
Dopp, Alex, 94
Drug Abuse Resistance Education
    (D.A.R.E.) program, 30, 141
Drug-Free Communities
    (SAMHSA), 103–4
Duckworth, Angela, 76–77
Durham Family Connects (Family
    Connects Durham), 47, 128
Dweck, Carol, 76–77

Early and Periodic Screening,
    Diagnostic, and Treatment
    (EPSDT), 125
Early Head Start, 41, 44

Early Risers, 62–63
EASEL (Ecological Approaches to
    Social Emotional Learning)
    Laboratory, 81, 82–83
EBIs (evidence-based
    interventions), 33
Ecological Approaches to Social
    Emotional Learning (EASEL)
    Laboratory, 81, 82–83
economic evaluation, 10–13
economics, 4–5
effectiveness
    of evidence-based
        interventions, 23–24
    ineffective programs, 21
    point estimate for, 23
Eisenberg, Daniel, 4–5
elementary school programs, 78
EPSDT (Early and Periodic
    Screening, Diagnostic, and
    Treatment), 125
equity
    assuring, 128
    considerations for, 50–51, 65–66,
        83, 99, 107, 111–12
evaluation
    economic, 10–13
    recommendations for frontline
        providers, 140–41
evidence, 18–20
    accessibility of, 133–34
    classifying and grading, 21
    incomplete, 21, 144
    lessons learned, 115–16
    need for better evidence, 115–16
    practice-based, 146
    recommendations for decision
        makers, 132–34
    recommendations for families,
        concerned citizens, and young
        people themselves, 147–48
    recommendations for researchers
        and funders of research, 144

types of, 22–24
usability of, 133–34
validity of, 22–23
evidence-based interventions
    (EBIs), 33
evidence-based policy, 19–20
evidence-based practice
    for children and
        adolescents, 1–2
    current evidence and
        practice, 18–36
    implementation of, 137–38
    practices vs programs, 98–99
    recommendations for decision
        makers, 137–38
    recommendations for frontline
        providers, 139–40
Evidence-Based Practices Resource
    Center, 33
experimental therapeutics
    approach, 145

faculty, 73–74
families, 147–48
Families First Preventive Services
    Act, 25–26, 131–32
Family Connects, 47–48
Family Connects Durham (Durham
    Family Connects), 47, 123–
    24, 128
Family Spirit, 51
family support specialists, 37
FDA (Food and Drug
    Administration), 144
feasibility, 23–24
feedback, 134
FFT (functional family
    therapy), 98–99
fifth grade programs, 15, 82–83
financing, 124–25
    pay-for-success, 92–93, 136–37
    recommendations for decision
        makers, 133–34, 136–37

recommendations for funders of
research, 143–47
wrong pockets problem,
91, 136–37
first grade programs, 82–83
flexibility, 132–33
focus power, 82–83
Food and Drug Administration
(FDA), 144
4Rs, 79–80
Franklin County and North
Quabbin Region
(Massachusetts), 111–12
Communities That Care (CTC)
coalition, 103–7, 123–24
Teen Health Survey, 104, 107
Franklin Regional Council of
Governments, 103–4
fraud, 96
frontline providers, 139–43
functional family therapy
(FFT), 98–99
funding. *See* financing
future directions
recommendations for better
investments, 131–49
recommendations for decision
makers, 131–39
recommendations for frontline
providers, 139–43
recommendations for researchers
and funders of research, 143–47
remaining questions, 114–30

Ganju, Vijay, 139–40
Generation Parent Management
Training-Oregon, 62–63
Germany, 107–8
Goggins, Lathardus, 71
Goodman, Benjamin, 47–48
Gordon, Eric, 70–71, 74–75
Greenberg, Mark, 75–76
Green Farms Academy (Bridgeport,
Connecticut), 82–83

grit, 76–77
growth mindsets, 76–77
Guidance Center (Wayne County,
Michigan), 94–96
Guiding Good Choices, 105

Haggerty, Kevin, 107–8, 109–10
*Handbook of Social and Emotional
Learning*, 78
Harrison, Bach, 108–9
Harvard Grant Study, 146–47
Hawkins, J. David, 107–8
health care providers, 139–43
health surveillance, 134–36
Healthy Families America, 38,
41, 44, 50
Healthy Families New York, 38
Heckman, James, 76–77
high school programs, 78, 82–83
Hill, Karl, 25
Hinton, Kim, 94
Hispanic Americans, 50–51
Home Visiting Evidence
of Effectiveness
(HomVEE), 40–41
home visiting programs, 37–54
active ingredients, 46
challenges in establishing and
preserving effectiveness, 45–46
core components, 46
economic case for, 49–50
equity considerations, 50–51
evidence of effectiveness, 42–44
flexibility and variation, 41–42
need for better evidence, 115
Horizons program, 82–83
Humanware, 71, 74–75

.Iceland, 136–37
implementation
continuum of, 142
deimplementation, 32–
33, 141–42
implementation science, 5

Incredible Years program, 58–59
  Advance curriculum, 59–60
  Basic curriculum, 59–60
  cost-effectiveness of, 63
  equity considerations, 66
  evidence of effectiveness, 62–63
  evidence of effectiveness and cost-
    effectiveness, 78
India, 127
individual champions, 123–24
infant mental health, 39
Infant Mental Health–Home
  Visiting, 39
infrastructure, 137–38
innovation, 148
intermediary/purveyor
  organizations (IPOs), 33
investment in children's
  mental health
  best investments, 10–13
  current practices, 29–31
  definition of, 8–9
  why we are not making good
    investments, 31–33
IPOs (intermediary/purveyor
  organizations), 33

kernels approach, 81–83, 118–21
Kerns, Suzanne, 92–93, 96–97
Kids Count, 134–35
kindergarteners, 15, 82–83

Latinx families, 65
LaVail, Renée, 97–98
leadership, local, 123–24
learning, social-emotional (SEL),
  12–13, 30, 70–85, 115
lessons learned, 114–30
Life Skills Training, 78, 79–80
Lipsey, Mark, 98–99
local champions and
  leadership, 123–24

Logan, Shelley, 109–10
long-term studies, 146–47

macro-culture, 65
Main, Denise, 132
Massachusetts
  Communities That Care
    (CTC), 103–7
  Franklin County and North
    Quabbin Region, 104, 111–
    12, 123–24
MATCH approach, 120
Maternal, Infant, and Early
  Childhood Home Visiting
  (MIECHV) program, 41, 43–44
McEachron, Cedric, 73–74
MDM (midday meal) program, 127
Medicaid, 5
  coverage for multisystemic
    therapy (MST), 91–92, 94–
    95, 96–97
  Early and Periodic Screening,
    Diagnostic, and Treatment
    (EPSDT), 125
  spending on, 49–51
Memorial Elementary School
  (Cleveland, Ohio), 71–72
mental health. See also children's
  mental health
  adolescent, 1–2, 9–10
  burden of disease, 2
  death rates, 1
  definition of, 9–10
  infant, 39
  recommendations for families,
    concerned citizens, and young
    people themselves, 148
Mental Health Technology
  Transfer Center (MHTTC)
  Network, 123
Mexico, 107–8
Michigan, 94–98

midday meal (MDM) program, 127
middle school programs, 78, 82–83
MIECHV (Maternal, Infant, and
    Early Childhood Home
    Visiting) program, 41, 43–44
mindfulness interventions, 78
Minnesota, 19–20, 138–39
Missouri, 46
Missouri Delinquency
    Project, 88–89
Morelli, Dorothy, 75–76
MOST (Multiphase Optimization
    Strategy) framework, 145
Mott Haven (Bronx, NY), 37
MST. See Multisystemic Therapy
MST Institute, 87
MST Services, 87, 88–89, 92, 121
Multiphase Optimization Strategy
    (MOST) framework, 145
Multisystemic Therapy (MST), 58–
    59, 86–101, 120
    benefit–cost ratio, 90–91, 136
    blended teams, 94
    core components, 119, 120
    costs, 89–93
    equity considerations, 99, 128
    evidence of effectiveness, 88–89
    financing strategies, 92
    implementation
        challenges, 93–94
    lessons from Michigan and New
        Mexico, 94–98
    Medicaid coverage, 91–92, 94–
        95, 96–97
    national penetration, 30, 98–99
    pay-for-success projects, 92–93
    telehealth adaptations, 98, 125

National Association of State Mental
    Health Program Directors
    Research Institute (rebranded
    as NRI), 137–38

National Child Abuse and Neglect
    Data System, 134–35
National Child Traumatic Stress
    Network, 137–38
National Commission on Social,
    Emotional, and Academic
    Development, 76–77
National Health Service (NHS), 63
National Incidence Study, 134–35
National Institute of Mental Health
    (NIMH), 137–38, 145–46
National Institutes of Health
    (NIH), 143–44
National Notifiable Diseases
    Surveillance System, 134–35
National Registry of Evidence-
    Based Programs and Practices
    (NREPP), 33
National Science
    Foundation, 143–44
National Vital Statistics
    System, 134–35
Navajo, 51
Network Partners, 87, 96–97
New Mexico, 138–39
    Children, Youth & Families
        Department (CYFD), 96–
        97, 136–37
    evidence-based policy, 19–20
    Human Services Department, 96
    lessons from, 94–98
new technologies, 125–26
New York State
    home visiting programs, 37–38
    Office of Children and Family
        Services (OCFS), 38
NFP. See Nurse–Family Partnership
NHS (National Health Service), 63
NIH (National Institutes of
    Health), 143–44
NIMH (National Institute of Mental
    Health), 137–38, 145–46

non-cognitive skills, 76–77
NREPP (National Registry of
   Evidence-Based Programs and
   Practices), 33
NRI (National Association
   of State Mental Health
   Program Directors Research
   Institute), 137–38
Nurse–Family Partnership (NFP),
   38, 39–42
   benefit–cost ratios, 49
   core elements, 119
   costs per family, 50
   economic evaluation of, 49–50
   equity considerations, 50–51, 128
   evidence of effectiveness, 42–43,
      44, 62–63
   national penetration, 30
   nurturing environments, 15–16

Ohio
   Cleveland Metropolitan School
      District, 70–76
   social-emotional learning (SEL)
      standards, 70–71
online tools, 126
online training, 110
oppositional defiant disorder, 86–87

parent–child centers, 55
parent–child interaction therapy
   (PCIT), 62–63, 64–65
Parent Effectiveness Traini0ng0
   (PET), 61
parenting interventions, 132
Parent Management Training
   Oregon, 66
Parents as Teachers, 41, 44, 46, 48, 50
parent training programs, 55–69
   behavioral, 59
   cost-effectiveness of, 63–64

disruptive behavior disorders
   and, 57–60
economic evaluation of, 63–65
equity considerations, 65–66
evidence of effectiveness, 61–63
need for better evidence, 115
nonbehavioral, 59–60
PATHS® (Promoting Alternative
   Thinking Strategies)
   curriculum, 71–74, 120, 123
   cost-effectiveness, 79–80
   evidence of effectiveness, 78
   implementation challenges, 80–81
   kernels approach, 83
   key ingredients for
      success, 74–75
   model schools, 76
   national penetration, 30, 80
PATHS Worldwide, 121
Patient-Centered Outcomes
   Research Institute
   (PCORI), 146
pay-for-success, 92–93, 136–37
PBIS (Positive Behavior
   Interventions and
   Supports), 80
PCIT (parent–child interaction
   therapy), 62–63, 64–65
PCORI (Patient-Centered Outcomes
   Research Institute), 146
PDSA (Plan-Do-Study-Act)
   cycle, 111
Penn State University, 28
Pennsylvania, 109
PET (Parent Effectiveness
   Training), 61
Pew Charitable Trusts, 28, 138–39
Pew-MacArthur Results First
   initiative, 27–28
Pierce, Craig, 96–97
Plan-Do-Check-Act cycle, 111

Plan-Do-Study-Act (PDSA) cycle, 111
point estimates, 23
population-focused approach, 47–48
population-level measurement, 134–36
Positive Action, 14, 78, 79–81
Positive Behavior Interventions and Supports (PBIS), 80
Positive Parenting Program (Triple P), 60, 62–63, 64, 66
postsecondary school programs, 78
post-traumatic stress disorder (PTSD), 86–87
practice-based evidence, 146
preschool programs, 78
preventive programs, 30, 124, 144
process improvement strategies, 111
Promoting Alternative Thinking Strategies. See PATHS
psychotherapy, 120–21
public health, 4–5
public health approach, 47–48
Public Health Data Modernization Initiative (CDC), 135
public health interventions
adaptable features, 145
core elements, 119–20, 145
deimplementation, 141–42
development of, 116–18
evaluation of, 140–41
financing, 124–25
new technologies for, 125–26
recommendations for better investments, 131–49
recommendations for decision makers, 131–39
recommendations for families, concerned citizens, and young people themselves, 147–48
recommendations for frontline providers, 139–43

recommendations for researchers and funders of research, 145
scaling up, 125–26
purveyor organizations, 121–23

quality-adjusted life year (QALY), 49–50

Raghavan, Ramesh, 5
Raising Healthy Children, 110
Rapid Response, 71
remember power, 82–83
research
long-term studies, 146–47
recommendations for researchers and funders, 143–47
remaining questions, 114–30
research evidence, 18–20. See also evidence
classifying and grading, 21
current evidence, 18–36
types of, 22–24
validity of, 22–23
residential placements, 86–87
Responding in Peaceful and Positive Ways (RIPP), 78
Responsive Classroom, 78, 79–80
Results First initiative, 27–28, 138–39
return-on-investment analysis, 10–11
Rodriguez, Amanda, 73–74
Rose, Geoffrey, 117

Sacramento, California, 81, 83
SAMHSA (Substance Abuse and Mental Health Services Administration)
Drug-Free Communities program, 103–4
Mental Health Technology Transfer Center (MHTTC) Network, 123

SAMHSA, (cont.)
   National Registry of Evidence-
      Based Programs and Practices
      (NREPP), 33
   Technology Transfer Center
      Networks, 137–38
Sanchez, Darmaris, 73
Say Yes program, 76
scaffolding, 15
scaling up, 125–26, 131–32
school-based social-emotional
      learning (SEL) programs,
      12–13, 84
   Cleveland Metropolitan School
      District, 70–76, 83
   equity considerations, 83
   evidence of effectiveness and cost-
      effectiveness, 77–80
   implementation
      challenges, 80–81
   kernels approach, 81–83
   key ingredients for success, 74–76
   national penetration, 30, 80
   need for better evidence, 115
   trends and lessons, 76–77
school nutrition, 127
school staff, 73–74
Scott, James, 18–19
SDS (Social Development
      Strategy), 110–11
Seattle Youth Development
      project, 110
second grade programs, 82–83
Second Step, 75–76, 78, 79–80
SEL. See social-emotional learning
SEL Worldwide, 75–76
Shea, Sage, 107
SNAP (Supplemental Nutrition
      Assistance Program), 49, 50–51
Social and Emotional
      Training, 79–80
social and emotional well-being, 8

Social Development Strategy
      (SDS), 110–11
social-ecological perspective, 13–14
social-emotional learning (SEL), 70
   kernels approach, 81–83
   need for better evidence, 115
   programs for teachers and other
      staff members, 73–74
   school-based programs, 12–13,
      30, 70–84
social impact bonds, 92
Social Programs That Work,
      25–26, 42–43
social vaccines, 118
societal perspective, 11
soft skills, 76–77
Southwest Family Guidance
      Center & Institute (New
      Mexico), 96, 97
SPEP (Standard Program Evaluation
      Protocol), 98–99
standardized programs, 118–21
Standard Program Evaluation
      Protocol (SPEP), 98–99
Stanford Social Innovation
      Review, 105–6
Stencil, Bill, 71, 74–76
Stepleton, Sue, 45, 48
Stoler, Rachel, 103–4
stop-and-think power, 82–83
Strother, Keller, 86
Substance Abuse and Mental Health
      Services Administration
      (SAMHSA)
   Drug-Free Communities
      program, 103–4
   Mental Health Technology
      Transfer Center (MHTTC)
      Network, 123
   National Registry of Evidence-
      Based Programs and Practices
      (NREPP), 33

Technology Transfer Center
Networks, 137–38
substance use disorders, 86–87
substance use prevention
programs, 30
Sunrise Family Resource Center, 55
Supplemental Nutrition Assistance
Program (SNAP), 49, 50–51
surveillance, 134–36
sustainability, 23–24
Sweden, 47–48, 107–8
synergy, 106

TANF (Temporary Assistance for
Needy Families), 49, 50–51
teachers, 73–74
technology
new technologies, 125–26
technology-based
communication, 94, 125–26
Technology Transfer Center
Networks (SAMHSA), 137–38
Teen Health Survey, 104, 107
telehealth, 97–98, 125
Temporary Assistance for Needy
Families (TANF), 49, 50–51
Title IV-E Prevention Services
Clearinghouse, 25–26
Tough, Paul, 76–77
treatment adaptation, 146. *See also*
adaptations
Triple P (Positive Parenting
Program), 60, 62–63, 64,
66, 128
Twin Rivers Unified District
(Sacramento, California), 81
two sources theory, 126

uncertainty, 23, 144–45
United Kingdom, 63
United States
evidence-based policy, 19–20

health surveillance, 134–36
United States Department of
Education, 133
University of New Mexico, 96–97
University of Washington, 107–
8, 109–10
Up!, 146–47
Urban Institute, 136–37
U.S. Department of Health and
Human Services (HHS)
Administration for Children and
Families (ACF), 25–26, 40–41
Home Visiting Evidence
of Effectiveness
(HomVEE), 40–41
Title IV-E Prevention Services
Clearinghouse, 25–26
U.S. Preventive Services Task
Force, 21
usability of evidence, 133–34
usual care, 139–40, 146

vaccines, social, 118
Vaillant, George, 146–47
validity, internal vs external, 22–23
Vermont, 55
Vermont Department for Children
and Families, 55
virtual communications, 97–
98, 125

Washington State Institute for Public
Policy (WSIPP), 3, 27–28
estimates of benefits of CTC, 109
estimates of benefits of MST, 90
estimates of benefits of parent
training programs, 63–65
estimates of benefits of SEL
programs, 79–80
feedback process, 134
funding, 133
Wayne County, Michigan, 94–96

What Works Clearinghouse, 133
"what works" registries, 25–28
white Americans, 50–51
Williams, Christopher, 81–82
World Health Organization
    (WHO), 9–10
wrong pockets problem, 91, 136–37

WSIPP. *See* Washington State
    Institute for Public Policy

yoga, 73–74
young people, 147–48
Youth Risk Behavior Surveillance
    System, 134–35